Rejuvenation of All Body Systems

Complete Guide
to
Whole Body
Cleansing

Information

Instructions

Self-Testing

By Dr. Yakov Koyfman, N.D.

The Great War
Inside You

When toxins come to a body,
the immune system begins
to fight them.
In counterattack, the toxins
link up with their best friends,
the parasites,
and use their most dangerous weapon,
poison.
This constant war leaves
the immune system tired and weak
and opens the door to diseases.
Killing the parasites and
cleansing the body from toxins
releases the immune system from its
major enemies.
The immune system becomes stronger
and health returns.

Preface

This book is published, not as a substitute for, but as a supplement to the supervision of a professional healthcare practitioner. The procedures described in this book are designed to support the body's immune system through internal cleansing so the body can heal itself and experience maximum vitality. They are preventative in nature for the improvement of human health. They are also designed to provide a greater self-awareness of personal health.

This book is not intended to provide medical consultation, diagnostic services, prognostication, or prescription for any ailment or condition. The author of this book does not treat any disease or provide any cure. Rather, this book is intended to offer information to help the reader cooperate with physicians and health professionals in a mutual quest for optimum well-being.

Because each person is unique, the author encourages each reader to pursue a daily self-care program tailored to his or her particular situation, based on that person's own best evaluation of the circumstances.

Koyfman Whole Body Cleansing
3107 Medlock Bridge Rd
Norcross, GA 30071
(770) 908-2305

www.koyfmancenter.com

Testimonials:

"... I do not need my **gallbladder surgery** *anymore. The stones have been flushed out of my system with only one Koyfman liver cleansing procedure..."*

Tracy K.

"...10 years of **severe sinusitis** *is gone after 6 visits with Dr. Koyfman, I can breath with my nose again..."*

Carrol D.

"... **Pacemaker** *is now out of question. My heart is better than it was 30 years ago. Water retention is gone. I ride my bike and run 2 miles a day at age 62. I am amazed..."*

Dan K.

"... just by taking his advice and using suggested natural remedies, **my thyroid started functioning noticeably better within one week.** *All I had to do, was some simple exercise, black radish juice and cleansing procedures. No more medication? It is great!"*

Diane T.

"... the **joints are not swollen and don't hurt.** *I forgot that feeling in 20 years. I thought nothing would change until I get to the actual joint cleanse, but I started feeling better with each cleansing procedure I did. His dietary and exercising advices are also great and simple..."*

Darren B.

* All testimonials in this book are real and true stories of healing told by our clients. However, to protect clients' confidentiality, their full names and contact information are not provided.

Contents

Prologue:

How to Use This Book

This book describes the techniques and philosophy that make up "Deep Internal Body Cleansing." This powerful suite of procedures is designed to help remove harmful toxins (chemical, biological, and mental) from specific organs and systems in your body. Once these disease-causing toxins are fully purged from the body, **maximum health is an attainable goal and a sustainable lifestyle.**

How to Use the Information

As you delve into each of the cleansing techniques recorded here you will find instructions on how to prepare and what to expect, what your part is and what the Center does. For example, as toxins are gently flushed from the body, some people sometimes experience minor discomfort as these toxins pass through the body on the way out. This discomfort is very temporary, but its possibility is important to know in order to understand "what's happening."

This book also provides information on what to eat to support your newly increased health.

Please read the instructions carefully, as they are vital to the success of these procedures. Do not skip any part of the instructions, and certainly do not neglect the whole of any one of them. It is recommended that you read each set of instructions several times to be sure you understand it correctly. Then either highlight or make notes of the basics of each step so you can remember what you have learned.

Please remember that the **"Trinity of Good Health"** is more than (1) eating correctly, (2) exercising properly, and (3) flushing toxins from the body. The Trinity of Good Health includes that most powerful of alliances: (1) correct knowledge, (2) a trained and experienced health care provider to guide you in the techniques, and (3) YOU.

Never underestimate the importance *you* play in all of this. It is not enough to merely "show up" for the procedures. You want to engage the knowledge you have and marry it to a focused commitment. When the power of the mind and the commitment of the heart are brought into play, all of the other elements of good health are given their greatest strength.

How to Use the Herbs, Beverages, and Solutions

All solutions which we use at the Center are completely organic, and made by hand by professionals for each individual. These solutions are made from fresh juices, herbs, minerals, and purified water.

All cleansings performed with these solutions require special preparation, and are based on knowledge acquired from centuries of practice. Professional experience and training are critical to the correct administration of these solutions to yield the maximum healing effect.

The contents of each of these solutions used at the Center, plus the techniques for properly blending the solutions, are proprietary information and are the intellectual property of the Center. Trying to duplicate these solutions at home can yield results that either interfere with or prove counterproductive to the cleansing procedures. Trying to fake these solutions can even be harmful since there are critical synergies involved with the components of the solutions.

Introduction:

Health and Cleansing

Healing through cleansing procedures is the easiest, quickest, and most natural way to get your health back. Cleansing is the best way, not only to heal problems, but also to prevent illness and maintain good health.

Cleansing

The most basic and undeniable concept in the health of the human organism is that "foreign" materials (things that were never meant to be part of the body) do **not** increase health. In fact, foreign objects *in any working system* (including mechanical) interfere with its proper functioning. (Scatter a handful of nuts, bolts and washers in the crankcase of an automobile and see what you get.)

The equivalent is true of our bodies. Unnatural chemicals and unwelcome biological agents (colds and flu, for example) interfere with the proper functioning of organs and systems, and use up the valuable resources of the immune system. Getting rid of these toxins paves the way for healing and prevention of illnesses.

Recently, many people have begun to understand this idea, and to popularize words like "cleansing," "detox," "detoxification," and other similar words and phrases. Each of these descriptions is partially true, but the real cleansing of the body is something very different and a lot more effective.

Awaken! It is not Too Late... Yet

Two processes of destruction and rehabilitation lead the fight in the human body from the moment of birth and to the end of the life. When we are young, the rehabilitation process is dominating where as process of destruction is still weak and not as significant. However, when we reach approximately thirty years of age (or even sooner) the destruction process grows stronger making the rehabilitation process weaker.

What exactly is being destructed in the body?

The cells of the body become clogged and overfilled with toxicity, loose their elasticity and begin to age. Skin and tissue stretch and hang. Joint glands clog-up and produce less lubrication causing joint bones to rub against each other. Gradually joints rub off and cover-up with salt crystals and uric acid. Polluted large intestine (colon) contaminates blood, blood vessels and lymph - slowing down circulation. The heart exhausts by trying to overcome the pressure in the colon and by pushing the blood through clogged-up vessels, and finally wears off. The energy drops drastically. Glands of internal secretion also become clogged. Lowers production and secretion of vital hormones. Slowly, but surely all organs and systems become congested and polluted, which significantly lowers their functioning. The body accumulates and produces more and more toxicity, and less nutrients to feed the immune system. The protection system weakens. Unfriendly bacteria, infection and other parasites meet less and less resistance from the immune system and reproduce easily. These creatures eat our nutrients, organs and muscles. They eat us alive! The body's resistance to destruction lowers rapidly and our unthoughtful actions speed up the process even more. The border line becomes closer and closer.

So how can you slow down that persistent stream of time and process of destruction?

Cleansing of the digestive system, liver, lymph and especially cellular cleansing (fasting)– are excellent methods to cleanse the body on the cellular level, which will stop the aging process. When cleansed on the cellular level, organs begin to rejuvenate their own functions, strengthen and reverse their age.

Also, by doing cellular cleansing, all organ functions go 10-15 or even more years back. You start feeling stronger and look younger. If you repeat it once in a while, illnesses and age will not be of your concern and you should have a healthy, functioning life until at least a 100 years. This is a real process of rejuvenation!

A Simple Test
To Determine the Toxicity Level
in Your Body.
Find out how strong your immune system is and how healthy you really are.

NOTE: Self-Testing is not a medical diagnostic. Self-Testing is an ability to listen and understand your body's language. If you learn to observe and understand your body's language, you will be able to detect and prevent many future disorders and illnesses on time.

Find out how strong your immune system is and how healthy you really are.

This test the most real information about the state of your health and the strength of your immune system. The test is simple and can be done any time of the day. Your energy levels constantly change during the day, so it would be very interesting for you to find out the strength of your immune system in the morning, evening, or when you're feeling weak or tired. You can easily test yourself anywhere. All that you would need for equipment is only clock or watch which show seconds.

General Information

Oxygen plays the main role in all processes in the body... It is food #1 for brain and cells; it is vital for proper and complete digestion as well as toxin neutralization, which accumulate in the system. More toxicity we have in the body-- more oxygen is used for it's neutralization-- less of it is left for other needs. Of course first of all, the body is trying to defend itself from toxins. Reduced oxygen levels in the

6

blood creates a perfect environment for viruses, bacteria, infections and other parasites to grow and multiply, and creating better environment for illnesses to be born.

Vice Versa... Less toxicity there is in the body--- more oxygen is accumulated in the blood--- least pleasant it is for parasites to live, meaning... less illnesses.
So, by testing how much oxygen is in your blood, means finding out how weak or strong your immune system really is.

Oxygen reserves in the blood can be determined by this simple test:

1. Sit down on edge of the chair. Relax. Back straight.

2. Breath normally. After a short exhale. Use your hand (whichever one is more comfortable) to hold your nose.

Hold your breath.

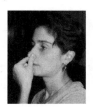

3. Hold it until first discomfort-- this is called **controlled pause.** Please do not confuse it with a **maximal pause!** Maximal pause is when you hold your breath to the maximum--it should be 2 times longer than controlled pause.

Time of the pause determine's how much oxygen you have in reserves of your blood, which at the same time determents reserves and strength of the whole body; its level of health and strength of immune system.

Here is a table to determine level of your health, illnesses and immune powers.

Length of the pause after exhale (Controlled pause)	Level of immune system	Illnesses level
less than 15 seconds	Immune system is very weak	know it or not, you have very serious illnesses
15 seconds	Your immune system is 4 time weaker than the norm	Your body already has some serious illness or you are very close to it.
30 seconds	Your immune system is 2 time weaker than the norm	Regular illnesses with a threat to become serious
45 seconds	immune system has 3/4 of the norm	Light illnesses not threatening yet.
60 seconds	Immune system is within norm	Rare, slightly noticeable problems
More than 60 seconds	Very strong immune system	No Illnesses or diseases

Other Methods of Self - Testing
to Determine Your State of Health and System's Disorders

Holistic medicine of the world created many different methods to detect all bodily disorders. To perform self-testing you are not required to have some deep knowledge of these methods. Many of the signs you already heard from your parents, grandparents, friends, books, or knew something from your own observations and experience. If you continue to observe, learn and develop your intuition, you will learn to feel your body, understand what it is asking for and what it is trying to teach you.

Determine your bodies ability to resist cancer.

Cancer cells always develop and grow in the human body. However, a healthy immune system immediately destroys and does not allow them to reproduce and grow into an illness. A simple method exists to determine your immune system's ability to resist reproduction of cancer cells.

It is best to do this test in the morning on empty stomach, or 2-3 hours before the test you may eat some kefir or plain yogurt. Meanwhile, take an **organic red beet**, wash it and peel the skin. Make 4 oz of juice from it and put in the refrigerator for 2-3 hours. Then, dilute that juice with 4 oz of filtered, room temperature water and drink the substance. Two to three hours after you drank the juice/water combination, collect your urine and look at its color. If the urine is light color or just a little brownish and cloudy-- your immune system is pretty strong and does not allow cancer cells to reproduce. If your urine is pink or red-- the immune system is weak and your body developed a good

9

environment for cancer cells to grow. You can strengthen your immune system through complete cleansing of your digestive system, liver and lymph cleansing, and if necessary-fasting.

So if you do have that predisposition, it is important to repeat this test once per month. If there is no suspicion to the problem, you may repeat the test every 3 months or more if desired.

What can your <u>SKIN</u> tell you?

Healthy skin does not have any irritations, pimples, boilers. It should be evenly colored, moderately moist, and feel good and firm to touch. Appearance of itching, pimples, painless or redness, increased dryness or oiliness, etc, indicates disorders.
For example:
Itching- allergy. Pimples/ boils-- increased toxicity.
Paleness-- anemia (lack of iron). Redness- impaired circulation, increased blood pressure. Dryness- dehydration.

Due to imbalances of the skin, lungs and kidneys, it might happen that the skin stops performing its cleansing function. In that case, lungs and kidneys get overwhelmed with toxicity, whereas the skin stays clean and does not send any signals of existing problems.

What does your TONGUE say besides words?

Determine your health with the help of your tongue. This test should be done first thing in the morning after awakening. All you need is a mirror. A healthy tongue does not have any coating. Its color is pink and even. Appearance of coating, change in color, cracks, increase of the tongues size, dryness, etc. suggest disorders in internal organs, especially in the digestive organs. Appearance of coating on the tongue- is a first signal, that digestive organs need cleansing.

Are you hungry?

Appetite is an important indicator of health or illness. A healthy appetite is a moderate need to eat simple, healthy products, which satisfy and fill the body. If the appetite is too strong- it might indicate irritation in the digestive system, such as gastritis, sugar imbalance in the blood or even parasites. If the appetite weakens- it might suggest indigestion or poisoning. Lack of appetite completely or disgust to food- is a sign of serious disorders in the body. In that case it is necessary to completely cleanse the digestive system, stop eating and wait for a real hunger.

Need more ENERGY?

A healthy body is full of energy and constant desire for doing, learning, and personal development. Reduction in energy, laziness, need for extra sleep-- are signals of increased toxicity. Your body is signaling you a warning of an illness. Complete lack of energy for a prolonged time, can be a result of stress, depression or some serious illness.

PAIN Language

Appearance of pain is a serious signal of bodily disorders. First signals tell about circulation disorder, accumulation of toxicity, exhaustion or physical disorder in the tissue and organs. Pain can also be caused by spread of infection in different organs.

SO...

As you can see, many methods can be used to determine what is going on in your body. I would like to provide you with more examples with the help of which you can determine your state of health. On purpose, I will not say what suggests health disorders and what means that you are in the good health. With time you will be able to determine which signal is good and which should warn you. Simple observation will teach you how to tell good from bad and will give you all the necessary answers. So observe and make your own conclusions. Some things to look for:

Your Stool: Dark, light, smell or no smell, light or hard, easily released or difficult, complete elimination or partial, regular (2-3 times per day) or not regular.

Saliva: Sticky, thick, dry, too much saliva or too little, no discomfort at all.

Hair: Thin, thick, falling off, dry, oily, hard or too soft, heavy or light.

Nails: Hard, soft, break easily, have white spots, ridges, moons on each nail or not, pink, dark, brutal.

Sweat: too much, too little, none at all, smell or no smell.

Urine: Dark, light, a lot, too little, often, rare, bad smell, no smell.

Sleep: deep, fall asleep easily, sleep all night without waking up. VS. waking up often, don't sleep enough, go to the restroom often. Wake up easily feeling rested and energized for the whole day, or tired wanting to sleep more. Dreams: no dreams, good dreams, nightmares.

Pulse: fast, slow, weak, strong, nervous, rhythmic, calm.

You can also use self testing by eyes, face lines, palms. You can use simple devices to measure blood pressure, temperature, pulse, etc.

Observe and memorize how you look when you feel good and full of energy. It will help you notice changes, which are different from your normal state of health. These changes will signal you of possible disorders and you will be able to take appropriate actions to prevent serious problems.

You can find more answers to your questions and concerns in my books "Healing Through Cleansing" volumes 1-4 and by coming to our center where our knowledgeable staff will be able to guide you in the right direction.

So, Do You Really Want to Be Healthy?

Physical, mental, and emotional energy are required to maintain good health, and even more so to regain good health.

Some people have spent 40 to 50 years ruining the condition of their bodies, and then think they can regain original health within a short time or in a few procedures. They are surprised when they learn that regaining health takes time, effort, energy, change of lifestyle, and healthy eating.

Stop for a moment and think this through. If it took decades to accumulate the poisons that are damaging your health, then it will take at least a little time to remove them. No, it won't take years to reverse the self-inflicted poisoning, but it will take time measured in months, maybe up to a year in severe cases.

The only way you can do it quickly is by the horrible path of surgery. Since toxins are often in all tissues down to the cellular level, can surgery even get them? No. It can remove gross contamination like accumulations in the colon, but at what price to your health? Do you really want to be put to sleep and then cut open to remove these poisons?

Often we hear phrases like, "I don't have time to do these cleansings." Here is something for you to consider.

Let's say that it took you an hour to travel to the Center, and hour in the office, and an hour to travel back home (or to your office). That is three hours. Now let's assume, for the sake of discussion, that you did this once a week for a year. That is 156 hours, or less than a week in terms of hours. Now compare that to the extra **years** of life you can expect because you cleansed your body from toxins. "Nuff said?"

A second consideration is to examine your day, starting with the morning and ending with the evening. Carefully think about each thing you do. Does everything you do have such important meaning to you that you cannot live without it? Is there anything as important to you as your health and life? I am sure that most people will find they waste lots of time on meaningless activities.

Examine your money in the same way. Who can say that he never bought things which he used one two times or never at all? Who can say that she bought only things that are necessary and really needed? Carefully look through your accounts and you will see how much you have spent for things that are meaningless or actually harmful. Get rid of these expenditures and invest in your health instead.

Famous author Neal Walsch claims that he has spoken with God. Once he asked God what to do to be healthy and live longer. God reportedly said, "You ask how to live longer but you, yourself, don't want to live longer." Neal affirmed that he really does want to be healthy, and God answered, "If you wanted to be healthy, you would not be smoking. If you wanted to be healthy, you would not eat meat of dead animals and other products which ruin your health."

Like the famous author, you need to evaluate whether really want to be healthy. To help you discover the strength of your determination, we offer you a test. In this test you need to mark, not the answer which you think is right, but the answer for which you are ready, the one you will do. Only then will you know for sure if you're determined to improve your health. Only then will you know which level of success you can reach.

Test Yourself to Determine How Strong Is Your Desire to Be Healthy

For each question, check (✓) all answers that apply:

1. In your opinion, what is the reason for your disease?
   - ☐ Genetics
   - ☐ Stress
   - ☐ Accident
   - ☐ Work in dangerous conditions
   - ☐ Other _____
   - ☐ Don't know

2. Whose responsibility is it that you are ill?
   - ☐ Your spouse
   - ☐ Friends or relatives
   - ☐ Your doctor
   - ☐ Your own laziness
   - ☐ Your unhealthy lifestyle and diet
   - ☐ Other _____
   - ☐ You don't know

3. Are you ready not only to do the cleansing procedures but also to invest your efforts and take your responsibility for your health?
   - ☐ Yes
   - ☐ No

4. The following are difficulties which may arise along your way. Which ones are you ready to meet?
   - ☐ Feeling worse before you get better
   - ☐ Staying on a plateau for awhile where nothing changes
   - ☐ Waking up 30 minutes or more earlier to walk and do other exercises
   - ☐ Refusing your favorite food:
     - ☐ Sweets
     - ☐ Meat
     - ☐ Ice Cream
     - ☐ Coffee
     - ☐ Other _____

5. Which of the following bad habits are you ready to quit or stay quit?

Quit	StayQuit	
☐	☐	Smoking
☐	☐	Alcohol
☐	☐	Drugs
☐	☐	Sitting for long periods watching television
☐	☐	Others

   _____

6. Are you ready to resist pressure from friends and relatives to break your chosen healthy way?
   - ☐ Yes
   - ☐ No

7. What effort are you ready to put out to get healthy?
   - ☐ A little
   - ☐ Moderate amount
   - ☐ Whatever it takes

8. How much money are you ready to spend to get healthy, that is for cleansing procedures, consultations, books, supplements, kitchen equipment, and health equipment?
   ☐ $75
   ☐ $300
   ☐ $1,000
   ☐ $10,000
   ☐ Whatever it takes

9. How much time are you ready to spend to get healthy?
   ☐ One week
   ☐ One month
   ☐ One year
   ☐ Whatever it takes

10. Which of the following is more important in your life than your health?
    ☐ Money
    ☐ Job or work
    ☐ Car
    ☐ Other _____
    ☐ Nothing at all

This test does not require score count in order to see if you really want to be healthy or have not yet recognized the importance of health to be happy and successful in life.

After you mark all the answers, you will easily see the level of your desire to be healthy. Although, just the fact that you have bought this book, means that the interest for your health already exists. If it is truly so, then the natural, internal cleansing techniques offered by our Center have a 100% potential to help you regain your maximum health and sustain it. To greatly increase your chances of success, you need to add to our work your conscious desire and efforts.

Healing Crisis

During the cleansing procedures provided in our center, 80 out of 100 people experience no unpleasant side effects. It is usually the opposite—with each cleanse, people feel better and better. However about 20% of our clients do experience an event of "Healing Crisis."

What is Healing Crisis?

Healing Crisis means—feeling worse before one can feel better.

The body of an adult person holds hundreds of different disorders. Most of them do not bother an individual at any given moment. However, "disorders" slowly worsen and get stronger, so that they can attack in the near future. Other disorders bother you once in a while, and you don't pay much attention. Only some disorders will constantly bother you, and those are likely the ones worrying you.

If, during the cleansing process, one begins to feel a disorder never felt before, it means that the **immune system was finally able to recognize it,** and that is great! You will feel worse and you might not like that, but now your body can begin the healing process. Understanding this should lift your spirits. Another piece of good news is that the "feeling bad" part won't last for too long. It might be a few hours or one to two days, rarely longer.

Why Should You Know about Healing Crisis?

If you know about the possibility of Healing Crisis, you won't be afraid if you should not feel well. On the contrary, now you'll understand that worse is the beginning of better! Remember, your positive thoughts and optimism are very important in your healing process.

Sometimes it happens that cleansing finds serious illnesses or disorders, which may have been there for many years growing stronger and waiting for the right time. If that is the case, then it might be recommended to consult your medical doctor to get the right diagnosis. In some cases it might be necessary to combine both traditional and alternative medicines. Don't be afraid to take medicine if you have to, because it won't be as harmful while you are going through the cleansing procedure, and it will help you kill the infection or bacteria so you can feel better and safe.

What Kind of Discomfort Might You Experience During Your Cleansing Procedures?

1. Colon Cleansing

It is, of course, hard to cover all possible discomforts, since everyone is different, but here are some common ones.

After the Colon Cleansing, you might feel bloating from the released gases and some sourness in places where you had gas pressure. You might see in the restroom a small amount of blood. This occurs because of some irritation and wounds on the walls of your large intestine after removal of hard fecal stones and parasites. Your hemorrhoids might flare up for a short period of time (even if you never knew you had them). Sometimes you might feel nausea, fatigue, headache, etc. Instructions in this book mention most of these problems and provide good explanation on how to ease them. If, in these instructions, there is no description of your discomfort or illness or problem, you must tell the Center's staff in order to receive appropriate advice.

2. Whole Digestive System Cleansing

If you are well prepared for this cleansing procedure you should not notice too much discomfort afterwards. However, in some people this cleansing procedure brings out impurity and clogginess of stomach walls with toxic mucus, bile, and undigested food. In this case, right during the procedure an intense cleansing might begin, possibly causing nausea or even vomiting which passes easily without straining or pain. Cleansing of the stomach walls will dramatically improve your digestion.

3. Complete Small Intestine Cleansing

During complete small intestine cleansing you might experience the same problems as during the Whole Digestive System Cleansing, although the chances of this are very small. After the cleansing you might feel tired, because the procedure is long and uses up a lot of internal energy. In this case, you should allow yourself to rest and be lazy for the rest of the day and go to bed very early to get more hours of sleep. You might also experience a release of negative emotions, which you can read about in detail in the books *"Deep Internal Body Cleansing"* or *"Healing Through Cleansing, Book 3."* Experiencing these inconveniences is a normal process that accompanies the cleansing of your small intestine. It is the beginning of some serious improvements and strengthening of your immune system.

4. Complex Liver Cleansing

Detailed description of discomfort during and after the Liver Cleansing is in the chapter "Instructions for Liver Cleansing." The better prepared you are, the less discomfort you will have.

5. Complete Lymph Cleansing

In very rare cases one might experience nausea, vomiting, or fatigue during Lymph Cleansing. An allergic reaction to citrus or carrot juices is also possible, even if you never had any problems with these juices before. During the Lymph Cleansing the quantity of produce consumed will be greatly increased and you might notice that you are, in fact, allergic to it. An allergic reaction might be in the form of itching skin, emotional instability, or something else. If that problem occurs, we will change the juice combination.

6. Sinus Cleansing

During the Sinus Cleansing, your system might find an infection in the mid-ear, which might start to ache. In order to exclude or lessen this discomfort, it is important not to blow your nose too hard during or after the sinus cleansing, since it might "wake up" the "sleeping" infection and activate it. If you completely cleanse your sinuses as well as your whole digestive system (colon, small intestine, stomach and liver), and remove the source of toxicity from the whole body, the infection will die on its own and will be flushed from the system naturally through the kidneys and colon.

7. Stomach, Joint, Cell and Other Cleansing Procedures
are described in detail in this book separately in their respective sections.

*** For more detailed information, please read Self-Testing sections for each cleanse.*

If you do not experience any uncomfortable reactions to cleansing procedures, you should continue in the regimen recommended to you by our Center's staff.

If you do have some strong reaction to the process, you might need to increase the time elapsed between your cleansing procedures in order to give your body more rest and time to recuperate. Do not overload yourself physically or emotionally. In any case, do not get scared of the cleansing process, and don't quit at the first sign of discomfort. The strong reaction only shows that you have a serious problem, and this reaction is your body's way to get rid of this problem.

Don't stand in the way of this opportunity.

Testimonials:

"...My gallbladder surgery was scheduled for today, but when I woke up in the morning, I realized that God could not give me an unnecessary organ to be removed. Since I moved to Jacksonville, FL, I was not able to see Dr. Koyfman on regular basis, but that morning, without any prep. or notice, I started driving. I called his center from the road and told him that I am all yellow, my gallbladder is overfilled with stones and I am driving to him to save me. It was risky for him, but he could not turn his back on me. They stayed with me until very late that evening trying to prepare me the best way possible for the Liver Cleanse. Next morning we all started early. It was a hard work for everyone trying to get those stones out of my system, but we did it! I passed three stones 4cm in diameter. It was painful. They massaged it out eventually. I could feel them moving through my small intestine. When I got back to Florida, I went for an ultrasound right away and was very happy to find out that my gallbladder was completely free of stones. My M.D. looked surprised and a little disappointed. I am very lucky to know about Dr. Koyfman and his center..." **Ronne M.**

"... After trying so many ways to lose weight (Weight watchers, different pills, personal trainer, different diets...), I gave up. It was all pointless. My weight did not change at all. When I came to Dr. Koyfman just to get a colonic I did not expect anything but to cleanse my colon. After just one colonic, my abdomen began to shrink and I decided to get on the Weight Loss Program. Two months later, I am 30 pounds lighter and look 15 years younger. My energy is great. Everyone who knows me is amazed how good I look. And I'm just enjoying all the complements I constantly get..."

Linda H.

"...I never even thought that at 50 I could feel better than when I was 20! After only a few cleanses I felt like I was dropping years. I exercise every day now. I can run and actually breath fine during it. My sexual performance is amazing. I feel like a teenager again or maybe better..."

Jonathan D.

"...I have never met a walking encyclopedia before. It is amazing how much Dr. Koyfman knows, how much training and experience he has. His books hold so much information and actual practical techniques, it seems like I could find an answer to any problem. His staff is also well trained and knowledgeable. I feel like they are my new family and I can't see my life without the Koyfman Center anymore".

Tracy C.

Our Center's

Unique Cleansing

Procedures

Description

Instructions

Self -Testing

Step #1

Colon Cleansing

"The essential foundation for personal health."

What Is Colon Hydrotherapy?

Colon hydrotherapy is a gentle, natural method of washing *long-term* wastes from the entire colon. When this is done, the body no longer has to deal with wastes accumulated during a lifetime, and can use more of its own strength to heal itself and fight disease.

Who Needs Colon Hydrotherapy?

Virtually everyone has these built-up wastes in the colon. Most people in developed countries eat a lot of processed foods. As these (unnatural) foods move through the colon, fluids are absorbed during the digestive process, and a very sticky waste is created. These wastes cling to the colon walls and rot, releasing toxins that the body has already rejected.

How Does Colon Hydrotherapy Work?

Colon hydrotherapy uses state-of-the-art equipment to gently introduce purified water into the colon. During a colon hydrotherapy session, the pressure and temperature are controlled by a trained and experienced colon hydrotherapist who stays right there with the client. The therapist keeps the temperature and pressure at comfortable levels based on the client's feelings and instructions.

Is Colon Hydrotherapy Safe and Sanitary?

Yes. Each client receives his or her own brand-new speculum and plastic hose, which are immediately disposed of after use. Since all water and wastes are completely contained in a closed system, there is no mess and no odor. The client's dignity is preserved by the use of private draping and room. The procedure is professionally performed and preserves modesty.

Is Colon Hydrotherapy Painful or Dangerous?

No. The pressure is less than that of naturally occurring gas. The most one feels is the urge to have a bowel movement. This urge is satisfied by the work of the constantly circulating water, which removes first the new waste, then the old, long-term wastes.

How Many Colon Hydrotherapy Sessions Does a Person Need?

It took a long time to build up the long-term wastes in your colon, so in order to remove them gently, it will take more than one session. Depending on one's personal health, level of toxicity, and desire to improve, a person might need ten to twelve sessions. After the series, a person might want to cleanse once a month.

Can Colon Hydrotherapy Affect the Flora Balance?

Good flora does not usually predominate in colons that have old wastes stuck to their walls. Colon hydrotherapy washes out, not only the bad flora, but also the environment in which it grows. Then good flora has the opportunity and ability to thrive in a clean environment.

Can Colon Hydrotherapy Affect the Electrolyte Balance?

Colon hydrotherapy has very little effect on the balance of electrolytes. The few that are lost are replaced by proper eating or by the fresh juices that you might drink later.

Can Colon Hydrotherapy Help to Control Weight?

Research from scientists in both America and Europe have demonstrated that people in the richer nations carry within their bodies anywhere from 10 to 50 pounds of accumulated toxic materials. Although this material is stored throughout the body, the majority of it is stored in the colon. Accumulated toxic waste materials slow down metabolism, beginning after age 25 or 30. Colon hydrotherapy helps a person to lose the toxic weight and to increase the metabolic rate at the same time.

Instructions
for
Colon Cleansing

Before Your Cleanse:

1. Don't eat or drink anything for **two hours** before the procedure. Those who'd like to lose weight, should stay on liquid diet for 12-24 hours.
2. For best results we suggest you not eat any foods that produce gases, such as beans, cabbage, cauliflower, broccoli, nuts, and bread, on the day the procedure will take place.
3. Avoid soft drinks on the day you'll have the procedure done. (In fact, avoid soft drinks altogether.)
4. For those who suffer from bloating, don't eat any raw fruits, vegetables or beans for 24 hours before and after the procedure. It is better to eat whole grains (brown rice, buckwheat, millet, quinoa, amaranth) steamed vegetables and freshly made vegetable juices.

After Your Cleanse:

1. If you have never had a colonic before, or haven't had one for a long time, it is much better if you have a colon cleansing 2 or 3 days in a row; this will help soften and eliminate hard clogs and colon stones, and it will also help eliminate a lot of gases, which may give you bloating and pain. Then you may continue the cleansing

once or twice per week. (The recommended number or frequency of procedures given upon individual considerations).

2. If you are too blocked and full with gas, it is normal to feel some discomfort after the procedure. If you experience pain or other problems that bother you, you may drink hot water (1 cup water plus 1 teaspoon lemon juice), 2 sips every 5 minutes, or put a pinch of sea salt under your tongue, until the salt is diluted. Then swallow the saliva and spit out any remaining salt grains. This helps to neutralize toxins, and you will start feeling better. If you need to, you can call us for consultation.

3. If you suffer from chronic hemorrhoids you may expect some discomfort in the rectum and sometimes a little blood. If you have chronic colitis, is possible that you may see some mucus with blood. If you have sluggish colon or suffer from constipation, after the cleansing you probably won't feel the need to have a bowel movement for 2 to 3 days. *When the Cleansing Program is completed you'll be rid of all these problems.* For your homework to help with this problem, read my book, *Healing through Cleansing, Book 3.*

4. To maintain a clean colon after you have completed a series of cleansings, it is recommended to go on a prevention program described in a later chapter of this book, entitled, "Maintenance Program."

5. Keep in mind that the toxins from the colon go first to the liver. When the liver becomes blocked they spread to other organs and systems, and clog blood vessels.

6. Keeping your colon clean can help you avoid many health-related problems, and also feel and look better, younger and more energetic.

7. To activate the cleansing cycle, it is recommended to follow a cleansing diet. See my book, *Deep Internal Body Cleansing,* chapter entitled, "Diet for Rational Health."

8. At the same time, in order to soften the toxic waste in the colon, it is a good idea to have a warm bath for 15 to 20 minutes, two to three times a week.

9. If, during the procedure you don't release a large amount of waste material and you feel discomfort, this is a sign that you are too blocked and your colon is weak. In this case, and in addition to the warm bath, you can put some castor oil compresses on the abdominal area. For this, follow the technique of the castor oil pack discussed later.

10. If, after colon cleansing, you feel cramping, it means that the water from the cleansing awakened the colon and activated peristaltic activity. The colon is now trying to push out the poisons which stick to its walls. Feelings of discomfort after the procedure mean that the muscle movements meet the resistance of blockages, hard and large masses which block the passages. The muscles are not able to overcome the resistance and break up the blockage, so they increase their tension, and this makes you feel cramping. As feces gathers and expands the space behind the blockage, you may feel some pain. Another possible reason for post-cleansing cramping is that one part of either the large or small intestine may be crossed over and constricting another part. To help the colon to break up the blockages and eliminate the mass of gas, it is necessary to do cleansing 2-3 or more days in a row, do abdominal massage, use the castor oil pack, take a warm bath, and drink a lot of liquid.

11. **To open more cleansing channels,** you can combine colon cleansing with FIR (cleansing from heavy metals), IOM (internal organ massage), infrared sauna, and full body cleansing massage.

Castor Oil Pack

1. Buy castor oil from a drug or grocery store.
2. Warm 4-8 oz. castor oil in a small jar or pan.
3. Cut a piece of sheet to size to cover the abdominal area all the way around to the sides.
4. Soak the piece of sheet in the warm oil and then spread the sheet over the abdomen.
5. Cover the sheet with plastic, maybe from a plastic bag.
6. Cover the plastic with a towel.
7. Apply moderate heat by hot water bottle or heating pad next to the towel.
8. Keep this castor oil pack in place for two hours.
9. Shower to clean the oil off.

It is better to do this castor oil pack on the day before Colon Cleansing.

Colon Cleansing is the basis of all cleansings and is included in other cleansing procedures, such as cleansing for kidneys, joints, parasites, and others.
Colon Cleansing relieves pressure in the abdominal area and creates a condition which works like a magnet for toxic biles, toxic mucous, crystals, stones, parasites and other toxic waste. All these poisons are drawn into the colon and then expelled.

Some Disorders and Illnesses Which Could Be Solved with Colon Cleansing

Constipation, gas, bloating, yeast infection, tiredness, skin problems, parasites, bad breathing, abdominal pain, depression, ...

Self- Testing
During and After Colon Cleansing Procedure

How you feel during the procedure, how well you cleanse while on the colonic table and how well you eliminate in the restroom after the procedure– depends on how well you are prepared. If during the procedure you suffer from cramps and gas, if the water is not going in well into your colon, or if you just can not wait until the procedure is over– it means that you did not follow all the dieting instructions before your cleanse; ate some gas forming foods (soy, beans, popcorn...), combined foods incorrectly (ate fruit with other foods for instance), or maybe you overate and/or ate close to your procedure. For best results, warmth around abdominal area is ideal (warm bath, heating pad, oil compress). Before each procedure, please carefully read the book *"Eight Steps to Perfect Health"* to prepare properly, and about food combining in the book 4 *"Healing Through Cleansing Diet"*. If you strictly follow all recommendations, you will be happy with the results of your cleanse.

If your procedure was unsuccessful, most likely, it was due to your poor preparation or an existing serious problem in your large intestine (constipation, parasites, gas, blockages, irritation, IBS, etc). Set your mind on patience and effort, since that's the only way to get better. Success comes to those who are ready to work and are not afraid of challenge.

What you may expect during your colon cleansing procedure?

Gas

You may notice an extreme amount of air bubbles in the tube of the machine. That means you have an accumulation of toxic gas in your large intestine. That gas accumulates in the digestive system creating pressure on other vital organs: lungs, heart, kidneys, and reproductive system, resulting in the malfunctioning of these organs. Pressure of gas and toxins on the walls of digestive organs can result in hernias and other serious problems.

A large accumulation of gas can be caused by wrong food combining, not chewing the food enough, bad quality foods, improper cooking technique, etc. All of these reasons create a great environment for growing harmful intestinal bacteria, which cause fermentation and decay resulting in an enormous gas accumulation in the digestive system.

If you consume foods, which feed the good bacteria, you receive nutrients to feed the body and strengthen your health. If you eat foods, which feed unfriendly bacteria and parasites, you will receive toxic gas. In order to get rid of gas, it is necessary to kill parasites, cleanse all of your digestive system from toxicity and start eating healthy.

Mucus

In the process of your procedure you may see a lot of mucus. That toxic mucus usually forms from undigested products (milk, cheese, ice cream...), white flour products (bread, pasts, pizza...), sweets (cakes, candy, cookies, chocolate...), overeating, etc. In the mucus always accumulates a large amount of microscopic bacteria, viruses and yeast. When mucus spreads through all organs it becomes a source of many illnesses– from colds to cancer.

Fecal Stones

Many people's large intestines are overloaded with fecal stones. Fecal stones are hard pieces of undigested and dehydrated foods (mainly proteins and starches). The combination of these two food categories cannot be digested properly and form stones if they are eaten at one meal. This traditional combination of proteins and carbohydrates takes away from your body 20-30 times more digestive energy, than when they are eaten separately. Weakening of your system– strengthens parasites and unfriendly bacteria, which steal nutrients from the food you eat and form fecal stones. Hardened stones can rub against colon walls creating irritation and even bleeding wounds, which may result in colitis, ulcers and other serious illnesses. In the weakened and wounded places can develop and grow parasites and fungus– causing polyps, diverticulites, IBS, and more.

Mucoid Plaque

During your first few cleanses, you may see long, black, rubber looking strings called mucoid plaque. It is a combination of undigested proteins, fats, carbohydrates, mucus and bile held together by dead and alive parasites, and their wastes. It becomes a breading ground for infection and viruses, which grow and spread throughout the body germinating different illnesses. The darker your toxic elimination is, the longer it has been in your colon.

Parasites

During your cleanse, in the tube of the machine, you may see alive and dead parasites, worms and yeast. There can be hundreds of different types of parasites living in the human digestive system (from microscopic, invisible to human eye bacteria to few feet long worms). So if you see a lot of mucus, it is a good indication of dangerous bacteria, infection, viruses and yeast being present as well. If you see short and long strings, it could be tapeworms, roundworms and many other dangerous type of parasites. Intestinal parasites destroy all digestive processes taking away important nutrients and eating your body alive.

If You are Overweight.

Overweight individuals have a perception that their organs are filled with more toxicity than of those who are of normal weight. So they usually expect to see a large amount of waste come out during the colon cleansing procedure. However, in some clients just the opposite happens. Why?

In people who are overweight, not only the outer body is increased in size, but internal organs as well. Internal organs of these individuals are filled with toxic wastes and are stretched out. As a result of that stretching, they take up more space in the abdominal cavity and press on each other creating blockages. The blockages can be so strong, that they might not allow the water to go in the colon properly. As a result, first 1-3 colonics might not seem very productive.

So if you are in the category of these clients, then in order to lower the pressure in the pressed organs and help dissolve toxicity, it is necessary for you to be on a liquid diet (water, juice, herbal tea) for 24 hours before each procedure and also warm up abdominal area as described in the "Preparation Instructions for Colon Cleansing".

Try not to get disappointed that not much comes out during your first procedures. Even by releasing gasses only, it lowers the pressure in the digestive organs and prepares you for the more successful cleansing during next procedures: Whole Digestive System and Small Intestine Cleanses during which you will eliminate the majority of wastes. Be patient and continue. Success comes to those who is not afraid of challenge and who do not give up.

Leaking on the Table.

In our practice, during the colon cleansing procedure, we often meet with a phenomena in which some client's anal muscle is so weak that it is unable to hold tightly the inserted speculum. As a result, during the procedure, water flows around the speculum onto the table. Weakened anal muscles can create other unpleasant accidents for an individual. With a sneeze, cough, or passing of gas, the large intestine may unexpectedly release fecal matter.

Why Does It Happen?

Accumulation of toxins and excess gas in the large intestine create enormous pressure on the rectum and anus. Straining in the restroom during elimination adds pressure on the vessels and anal muscles. As a result, vessels in that area expand and push out through the muscle tissue (called hemorrhoids), and also the muscle itself becomes weakened.

Eastern medicine believes that by the strength or weakness of the anal muscle, you can diagnose the biological age of a person. The weaker anal muscle is, the older the person is biologically. This means that 35-year-old person with a weak anal muscle could have a biological age of 65-70, and vice versa. If an elderly individual has strong anal muscles, his or her biological age may be 20-30. Anal muscles can be strengthened by cleansing, exercise, and self-massage, as described in my book *"Healing Through Cleansing 3"*. By doing this exercise regularly, it will not only free you of discomfort associated with a weak anus, but also improve your sexual performance, rejuvenate your whole body and reverse your age.

Self-Test after procedure, while in the restroom.

If your colon muscles are weak, you will not be able to eliminate much on the colonic table, because you are in the laying position (which is not a natural position for elimination). In that case, with the help of gravity, you should have a good elimination in the restroom right after your procedure. If you would look in the toilet and check your elimination, you would be able to see everything described earlier. Although, sometimes the waste can be very thick and dark, which would make is difficult to see anything. However, that darkness, thickness and a horrible smell, can tell you a lot about what you have been keeping inside.

Just water?

There might be a case that during your procedure you absorb a lot of water, but it comes out very light colored or clear. Some blockages or other issues could be the reason. Because the water stays in the colon for a prolonged time, it has a chance to dissolve most of the blockages so when you go to the restroom after your procedure, you may release water of dark color. Some people after using the restroom, say that nothing but water came out. It is a wrong assumption. That colored water is a dissolved toxic waste.

That water does not have any hard matter, it was all dissolved into toxic cocktail. So the cleanse was still a success!

Leaky Gut– a result of toxins and gas, which stretched and damaged the colon walls making them too thin causing leakage of toxicity into the system.

If you suffer from leaky gut syndrome, a part of the water absorbed by your colon, may be absorbed into your blood stream. If it does happen, you may feel some tiredness, headache or some other discomfort. There is nothing to worry about. To neutralize that toxicity a lower its concentration, drink more hot water with lemon or herbal tea (chamomile or dandelion root). So in order to get rid of the root of the disorder- cleanse your digestive system completely, follow good diet and regularly perform exercises #6 and #7 from the book "Unique Method of Rejuvenation".

Smell

That bad, toxic smell is a smell of your illnesses and diseases, which destroy your body. If that smell is so strong in the open space of the restroom that you have to use an air freshener, think how horrible it is for the closed space of your small body, your organs and blood when it is constantly inside.

Sticky stool

Something else you should pay attention to in the restroom. If after you flush the toilet, it is left stained from your stool and you have to use the brush to scrub it off, it indicates an excess amount of undigested toxic fats in your stool and it sticks the same way to the walls of your colon, rectum and blood vessels. That is where the bad cholesterol comes from resulting in high blood pressure, heart and cardiovascular disorders.

Does it sink or float?

Another thing to look for. Your stool is supposed to sink. If it floats on top, it means that it is filled with gas, yeast, mucus and infection.

Hemorrhoids

In vary rare cases, after colon cleansing, you might get and "open hemorrhoid", which may start hurting, itching or bleeding. If you never knew about it, it means that it was internal and you never felt it. In that case, cleansing dragged it out, before it could develop into something more serious. Until that moment, neither you nor your body, tried to fight it. You did not even know it existed. Now that the problem is recognized, your body can start a healing process and you can help with your own efforts to help it (please see the book *"Unique Method of Colon Rejuvenation"*).

What if nothing came out?

There is also a possibility that nothing or not much will be eliminated even in the restroom after your procedure. Do not be disappointed. The number one reason for that happening is dehydration. Dehydration could be caused by not drinking enough water or because your body is not able to store water due to too much toxicity. Dehydration would make the waste in your colon very dry and it would absorb all the water like a sponge. Because of that, it would take sometime to soak, dissolve and be soft enough to be released. In that case we strongly suggest that you come back for another colon cleansing as soon as possible, preferably the next day, to not allow it to harden up again.

Conclusion

During each cleansing procedure, pay close attention to what you are eliminating and make your conclusions accordingly. **What do you carry inside? How it accumulated there? What you can do to cleanse your internal environment and not let it reoccur?**

If you really want to be healthy, internally clean and not know illnesses, you should:

1. Eat right
2. Lead a Healthy Life Style
3. Periodically, cleanse your system throughout the whole life.

SELF HELP: *CONSTIPATION*

If you suffer from constipation you have to learn special techniques to strengthen the muscle of your large intestine from my book "Healing Through Cleansing 1". Also try one of these simple recipes.

- *Cut up 2 medium size apples with skin (washed well from wax) to very small pieces. Put it in the pot and add 1.5 cups of milk and ½ cup of water. Bring to a boil and cook for 5 minutes. Take in the morning on empty stomach as breakfast, eat the apples and drink the liquid.*

- *Drink 1-2 cups of Freshly squeezed vegetable juices, mainly carrot + spinach, as well as others: beet + apple, carrot + celery, etc... 20-30 minutes before lunch and dinner.*
- *Drink 1 tablespoon of sunflower oil every hour until the colon begins to work. Use 1-2 times/week. Everyday you can drink 1 tablespoon on empty stomach first thing in the morning.*

Testimonials:

"... I have suffered from constipation all of my life. Dr. Koyfman told me that I would need more than just colon cleanses to get rid of my problem, but I was amazed to see that even after my first procedure I felt so much better! I felt light and clean. I was even able to go to the restroom on my own without any laxatives or any other help. His staff is great and very knowledgeable. I can't wait to feel even better..."

Tina K.

"... I was so clogged up that during my first 3 colon cleanses nothing would come out during the procedure. After the cleanse, I would spend 40 minutes in the restroom releasing all the toxins I have saved up. At first I was disappointed that nothing would come out during the procedure itself, but I felt so much better after each cleanse, that it didn't really matter. On my fourth colonic I say huge worms come out, one after another and ever since then my colonics were much more successful. I fell like a new person..." Larry B

Step #2

Whole Digestive System Cleansing

"Should be the cleanest place in the body."

Cleansing the whole digestive system in one focused effort will release the body's energies for use in more important matters.

Why Is Colon Cleansing Not Enough?

Colon Cleansing is a powerful procedure which eliminates toxins and parasites from the large intestine, and greatly improves its function of the colon and the well being of the whole body.

Unfortunately, many people have colons that are in such poor health that its malfunctioning undermines the whole digestive system. Once this starts, a badly impacted colon results in poor digestion that affects the whole digestive system. This causes the colon to be more severely impacted. It is a viscous circle.

So it is important to cleanse and improve the function of all the organs which are involved in digestion: stomach, pancreas, liver, and all parts of the small intestine. When we cleanse the digestive system from toxicity, it stops poisoning the body and improves its nourishment.

The Kitchen of the Human Body

The digestive system is one of the main channels through which nutrients enter the body. At the same time it is also the main elimination channel. An improper and unhealthy lifestyle transforms the digestive system from a source of nutrients, energy, and health into a source of toxicity, parasites, and illnesses.

The digestive system is the kitchen of the human body, and as such should be the cleanest place in the body. Instead, it becomes like a sewage holding tank full of poisons.

On the positive side, the digestive system is a unique set of organs which has a door on each end. Because the whole body is interested in nutrients, the digestive system has connection with all organs and cells through blood vessels, lymph, and various ducts. These facts present a unique opportunity not only to cleanse and improve the digestive system but also to use it as the main elimination channel through which to cleanse many other organs from toxicity and parasites.

Notice: Details of how to cleanse the whole digestive system will become familiar to the client during the individual consultation.

44

Why Is It Important to Keep the Digestive Tract Clean?

The digestive system is the "kitchen" of the human body in that it provides the food or nutrients our bodies need to live. How we keep that kitchen determines whether we will be feeding ourselves with nutrients or poisoning it with toxins.

Those who are truly interested in maintaining their health know the importance of cleaning the kitchen, as well as the continuing importance of maintaining it by regular cleansings.

No matter how good your diet, in our poisoned world you cannot completely keep toxins out of your body, hence the need for regular cleansings. Toxins not cleansed from the digestive system are absorbed into the blood and lymph systems, spread all over the body, and poison every organ and tissue down to the cellular level.

The immune system, weakened by this toxicity, first grows sluggish and less effective and finally becomes overwhelmed and surrenders. When it collapses, almost every disease can do its worst in your body.

In our Center we utilize a full spectrum of cleansing procedures. One of the simplest and most effective procedures is one I recently created, called "Whole Digestive System Cleansing ©." Our clients like this procedure because it is exactly that: simple and effective.

In one case, a woman completely stopped her migraine headaches, from which she had suffered for five years. This she did in only three procedures.

In another interesting case, one woman suffered from constant fatigue and muscle pain. Her blood test was seriously abnormal showing life-threatening factors. After

45

eight weeks of doing the Whole Digestive System Cleansing©
each week, she started feeling a surge of energy which she
has not felt in years. The pain in her muscles disappeared,
and the primary amazing result was that her blood test
became ideal.

Whole Digestive System Cleansing© is also helpful
when combined with other cleansing procedures, increasing
the effectiveness of each one. All these procedures,
preparations, and performances are described in detail in this
book.

Therapeutic Benefits of Cleansing the Whole Digestive System

- Cleanse and improve stomach function
- Cleanse and improve pancreas function
- Activate the liver
- Partially cleanse and improve the function of the small intestine
- Cleanse and improve the function of the colon
- Cleanse waste from the walls of the whole digestive system
- Eliminate a bad smell from the skin, breath, urine, and bowel
- Eliminate toxic gases
- Activate nerves, digestive buds
- Dramatically improve digestion

Short List of Disorders Which Could Be Helped with this Cleansing

Constipation, Poor Digestion, Chronic Fatigue, Diabetes, Obesity, Chronic Colitis, Chronic Appendicitis, Headaches, Poor Sleep Patterns, Skin Disorders, Sexual Disorders.

SELF HELP: *GAS AND BLOATING*

If you have a lot of gas and bloating switch to a monodiet for 2-3 days, up to a week. Monodiet means you eat only one product either in one meal or for the whole day (more effective). So you can choose to eat only brown rice or only cucumbers, etc... For details on different diets, see my book #4 "Healing Through Cleansing Diet"

If you suffer from yeast, reduce consumption of sweets and fats in your diet. When you eat fruit, only eat one type of fruit and on empty stomach. Perform breathing exercises from my book "Healing Through Cleansing 1" (colon chapter) and self-massage from "Healing Through Cleansing 3".

Instructions
for
Whole Digestive System
Cleansing

Preparation for Cleansing the Whole Digestive System

Before Cleansing the Whole Digestive System, do not eat for 6-10 or more hours. (For those who want to lose more weight, who have a sluggish system, or who have constipation, a liquid diet for 24-36 hours is a must). Your last meal should be light and of a small amount. Avoid meat and foods which produce gas for 1-2 days before the cleanse. **For more details, review the instructions for Colon Cleansing.**

What Should I Eat During the Cleansing Procedure?

Diet plays an important role in maintaining health. At the same time, a healthy diet is an agent of cleansing, nourishing, and healing.

Important principles of healthy eating, simple recipes, and weight loss programs are described in Book 4 of my series, *Healing through Cleansing Diet.*

Self-Testing
During the
Whole Digestive System

The Whole Digestive System cleansing procedure will partially cleanse your digestive tract (stomach, small intestine and colon) and flush out toxic accumulations and parasites from these organs through your bowels.

Pay Attention, Notice, Concentrate

When you start eliminating in the restroom, during your cleanse, you may not see a pretty picture. However, it should not make you turn away from it and flush the toilet without looking. It is important to investigate it. Pay special attention to the color, form and structure of the elimination. Look for parasites as well. Pay close attention to the smell of what you've been carrying inside for years; what sounds it comes out with. All these things are worth noticing and thinking about. Think of connection between what you eat and what comes out of you. Try to understand what kind of damage is being caused to your health by fermented and rotted waste inside of you. Think what it can do if you continue accumulating and carrying that dirt inside of your digestive system.

Notice how much lighter your body feels after you eliminated only a part of that "dirt". Think how great you will feel after you completely remove all the waste from your whole body and will begin to eat and live following principles of nature.

Cleansing Your Stomach

Whole Digestive System cleansing is a good alternative for stomach cleansing if you don't have a good vomiting reflex or vomiting itself scares you. This cleanse is gentle and not at all straining. In some cases, during the first W.D.S. cleansing, people feel nauseous. That is a sign of high toxic accumulation in the stomach and blockages in the small intestine, which are not allowing the solution to go down. If you are not scared to vomit, drink 1-2 glasses of your solution very quickly, go to the restroom, put two finger in your mouth and press on root of the tongue. Your stomach will easily release the toxicity, nausea will be gone, the solution will partly get into the small intestine and dissolve the blockage, and you will be able to continue the procedure without any problems. If you are afraid to vomit, drink your solution very slow and try to move (don't just sit) and massage your stomach lightly trying to push the solution down. You should not experience the same problem during your second W.D.S. cleansing.

Good Combinations

Whole Digestive System cleansing can be combined with other cleansing procedures, which will make it even more powerful and effective. You may choose to combine it with: Thyroid, Kidney, Prostate or Lung Cleanses. To do that, we put FIR (far infrared rays) on those organs. FIR penetrates deep into the organs on the cellular level, dissolves toxicity and expands pathway for elimination.

Mineral solution which you drink during your W.D.S. Cleanse, not only cleanses and disinfects the digestive system, it travels through the whole digestive tract and works as a magnet- attracting toxins dissolved by the FIR. When that toxicity gets into the digestive system, it is being flushed out (through the colon and sometimes kidneys) together with other "dirt", which has been there for years.

Whole Digestive System cleansing is great in combination with FIR Sauna. Especially this combination is great for those who have weak kidneys or a Leaky Gut Syndrome. With these problems, parts of dissolved toxins can be absorbed into the bloodstream and tissue, creating water-retention. By combining this cleanse with the FIR Sauna, all that absorbed toxicity is being eliminated through open pores of the skin. This process would also ease and improve working ability of the kidneys.

The Whole Digestive System Cleansing will prepare you for the Complete Small Intestine Cleansing.

"... What an amazing cleanse! So gentle and effective. I am so glad I had the guts to do it. For the first time in many years, after this cleanse, I ate and did not feel fool after only a few bites. I did not get my regular gas and indigestion after the meal and I am so grateful to experience it again. And the best thing is that, the good feeling is not going away, it is only getting better!"

Amy R.

Step #3

Small Intestine Cleansing

"Establishing healthy flora for normal digestion."

The Small Intestine as the "Abdominal Brain"

The small intestine is that part of the digestive tract between the stomach and the large intestine. It is one of the largest organs in the human body, and in adults can be as long as 30 feet. Together with the colon, it makes up the abdominal cavity.

The small intestine takes over where the stomach left off, further digesting the food eaten. Bile is mixed with the partially digested food to increase the effect of pancreatic juices that break down fats.

Although children may refer to this area of the body as the "tummy," in the East it is referred to as the "abdominal brain." This is because this intriguing organ not only digests food, but it also "digests" emotions.

52

The many different negative emotions are stored in very different but specific parts of the small intestine in the form of constrictions and curves. For example, anger tightens the right part of the small intestine near the liver. Nervousness affects the upper left part of the small intestine under the spleen. Impatience and anxiety affect the middle of the upper portion of the small intestine, while sadness attacks both sides of the lower parts. Fear, as may be expected, reaches into the deep lower parts.

On a physical level alone, the small intestine is vulnerable to another concern, and that is the long-term accumulation of wastes that build up due to incomplete digestion. These wastes line the small intestine and basically form a toxic layer that releases toxic chemicals into the bloodstream. These slowly acquired wastes also form an optimal environment for parasites to grow.

When the small intestine is overloaded with such toxins, it slows down the digestive process, and decreases its absorbing function. In this situation a person can eat large amounts of food and still be undernourished.

If the small intestine is overloaded with toxins, it loses its natural *tone* and begins to expand. (In fact, some of the large "bellies" you can see are a result of this.) This now larger and heavier organ puts pressure on other, underlying organs in the abdominal cavity and harms their health. Pressure on the veins interferes with circulation and can lead to varicose veins and hemorrhoids. In women, it can lead to menstrual disorders.

The extra weight of the unhealthy small intestine can even begin to pull on the spine, causing various back problems. This in turn can affect the diaphragm and cause imperceptible breathing difficulties.

An unhealthy small intestine increases the production of mucous in the lungs making sinus conditions more troublesome. Even the lymphatic system is impacted by an unclean small intestine.

Combine a physically unclean small intestine with long-term stored negative emotions and one sets the stage for bad health. This is why it is so very important to have a healthy small intestine. The best way to achieve this to practice a proper diet combined with **cleansing** this important organ of long-term wastes that have accumulated over a lifetime.

At the Koyfman Center we have a natural, gentle method of cleansing the small intestine. Based on centuries-proven techniques, the Center can help the body discharge this unwanted waste so that digestion will be improved, and so that the body will not have to spend precious energy fighting the toxins that come from this waste. Overall health will be improved by a strengthened immune system. This will help with the release of the negative emotions that are also stored in this vital organ.

Testimonial:

"...Having a severe yeast overgrowth is not fun at all. Constant yeast infections, antibiotics from doctors, creams and other junk to treat it felt endless. Nothing ever helped and only made it worse. Only through Dr. Koyfman I found out that yeast is actually an intestinal diseases. During my first Small Intestine procedure I saw so much yeast come out, it was unbelievable. I kept my diet strict for a few days and felt amazing since than! No more gas, bloating, vaginal yeast, brain fog, fatigue. I cannot believe it was all do to that small parasite..."   *Debbie K.*

Instructions
for
Small Intestine
Cleansing

Cleansing from Parasites, Yeast, and Heavy Metals

During the Whole Digestive System Cleansing© in our Center, we partly cleanse the small intestine from toxicity; however, the walls of the small intestine are still covered with a thick layer of sticky toxic mucus wherein reside many unfriendly bacteria and parasites.

Because the small intestine carries many nutrients, it attracts many parasites, bacteria, and yeasts to reside there. Parasites which live in the small intestine try to stay closer to the walls in order to steal more nutrients through contact with the blood, and in order to avoid being ejected. Toxic mucus not only sticks to the walls of the small intestine but also seeps inside those walls.

Next, on the walls of the small intestine there accumulate a lot of toxic bile and poisonous heavy metals. Because the small intestine is an organ of absorption, part of these metals' poisons absorb into the blood and lymph, going to the liver, glands, and even the brain. When toxic metals reach the brain, they destroy brain circulation and can cause memory loss and foggy thinking and many other problems. To flush out this sticky mucus; and eliminate all parasites, yeast, and poisonous heavy metals from the small intestine is not so easy. The only procedure able to do that effectively is the Small Intestine Cleansing© which was created in our Center. After the first procedure, with clean walls of the small intestine, the solution you drink will work like a magnet and will pull toxins and heavy metals from the blood vessels and lymph through the wall of the small intestine and will flush it through the same channel, the small intestine and the colon.

To get the best results from this procedure, it is necessary to start eating right, to do a Parasite Cleansing, to start taking friendly bacteria orally and by implantation directly through the rectum, repeating Small Intestine Cleansing 2-5 times and in some cases even more.

Preparation

For two to three days before the procedure, follow a vegetarian diet of foods that are rich in fiber: fresh fruits and vegetables, whole grains, dried (and soaked overnight)fruits, nuts and seeds.

Then 24 hours before the procedure, begin juice fasting. Those who need to lose weight may fast 36-48 hours. This means that the only food you will have is freshly made juices from carrots or other vegetables, water and herbal teas.

For those who have yeast problems, it is better to avoid sweet juices and drink green juices from cucumber, celery, spinach, etc., with 30-40% apple or carrot juice for taste. Grapefruit juice is also acceptable.

During this 24 hours, one should drink 1-2 cups of these fluids approximately every two hours during the day to maintain energy. This will also alleviate hunger. Laxatives and enemas are not recommended.

If you suffer from constipation and your colon doesn't eliminate its waste every day, you must have a colonic three days before the procedure. It would also be beneficial to take a warm bath for 15 to 20 minutes one day before the procedure. Please wear loose-fitting clothes that do not constrict your circulation or movement in the large intestine. The loose clothing is also appropriate since you will be doing some **mild** exercises.

Performing the Procedure

The cleansing of the small intestine can be done only on an empty stomach.

Performing the procedure includes:
- Drinking a natural, organic solution (liquid) that is prepared and provided by the Center.
- Performing some very mild "exercises" under the direction of Center personnel trained in this procedure.
- Receiving different types of help to allow the solution to freely move through the digestive tract.

The above procedure will stimulate the entire digestive tract to eliminate waste. At first you will eliminate regular feces. Then the elimination will become more watery. **Our goal is to expel liquid with the same color and consistency as the solution you have been drinking.**

After the procedure you will receive a meal of carefully cooked brown rice (or other whole grain) without salt or other spices. We add only Ghee (clarified butter) to this. You are allowed to eat only 7-9 ounces of rice or less, even if you are still hungry. You need to chew your meal slowly and properly, trying to chew every mouthful 50 to 100 times. **If you are using this procedure to begin a fast, you will not receive this meal.**

After Your First Meal

One or two hours after your first meal you may drink spring or distilled water. You may also drink chamomile or mint tea, with no sweeteners.

For lunch you may choose another grain meal, with well-steamed vegetables (carrots, onions, celery, etc.) and Ghee or cold pressed olive oil. In this meal you may add, if you want to, a little sea salt.

Do not eat raw vegetables or fruits, dairy products, meat, or spices. On the first day, even if you are a raw foodist, it is better not to eat any raw vegetables or fruits. **It is necessary to strictly follow this eating program for at least one day!**

Diet for the Days Following the Cleansing of the Small Intestine

On the next day, you may go back to your regular diet. For those who have been suffering from bloating, or if you have candida or other digestive problems, it is important to establish a healthy environment in the digestive tract. This includes proper conditions for the development of friendly bacteria whose natural job is to promote good digestion.

With this goal in mind:

1. Eat cooked vegetarian food for 3-5 days.
2. Follow the proper food combining rules. (Provided by the Center.)
3. Take acidophilus orally and through the rectum with a special syringe.
4. Don't eat sweets, or even honey.
5. After the period of eating only cooked vegetarian food, then eat lots of garlic and onions for at least 3-5 days.
6. Properly chew your food. This will help you release lots of saliva, which has disinfectant and cleansing properties.

Suggestions and Explanation for the Cleansing of the Small Intestine

1. Sip the solution. Do not rush, and don't drink too slowly. The drinking speed for one cup is approximately 1-3 minutes.
2. On the day of the small intestine cleansing you will likely feel tired and relaxed. This is normal because you are spending lots of energy getting rid of poisons and negative energy that was in your digestive system. If you need to, you may rest and sleep after the procedure. Please don't plan too many activities for the rest of the day after this procedure. In fact, you might consider planning to read a book or some other relaxed activity. After the Small Intestine Cleansing, you may feel relaxed and cheerful or experience a release of negative emotions collected in your gut.

3. ***Before*** the procedure, the digestive system is usually overloaded with food, and creates pressure on the surrounding organs. ***After*** the Small Intestine Cleansing, practically the whole digestive system is completely empty, creating a mild negative pressure. To fill the digestive system again after your have resumed eating normally takes 24-36 hours, perhaps more. **During this time, the negative pressure created by an empty digestive system intensively pulls toxins from the other organs.** (This is actually a change in "toxic pressure" causing toxins to migrate to the area of low toxic pressure, the small intestine.) This means that in 2-5 days after this cleansing, the small intestine will likely accumulate a large amount of toxins. This sudden influx of toxins (not food) creates a noticeable change in this organ. You may begin to feel some discomfort. These toxins will naturally move to the large intestine. Therefore, it is recommended that you do a Colon Cleansing during this time to help the body to get rid of these toxins.

4. The time from your first meal to your first bowel movement is a real transition time for the digestive and elimination systems. If this time is more than 36 hours, it indicates weak digestion and constipation. This is valuable information in that it gives a clearer understanding of an underlying condition in your digestive system.

5. To eliminate parasites and their eggs, to get rid of yeast, and to improve digestion, it is recommended to repeat the cleansing of the small intestine four or five times, leaving a break of two or three weeks in between. When you reach your goal, and to maintain this good level, you can repeat this procedure once or

twice a year, or more often if your particular situation calls for it.

Re-Colonizing Friendly Bacteria

Small Intestine Cleansing creates optimal conditions for the development of friendly bacteria. First it removes toxins and other negative environmental conditions that make it difficult for friendly bacteria to thrive. Secondly, it creates a healthy environment for the establishment and maintenance of friendly bacteria.

The best re-colonization results occur when the re-colonizing of friendly bacteria comes from two directions, through the mouth and through the rectum. To implant friendly bacteria into the colon, we use a special "syringe" with a two-ounce volume. Be assured that this syringe does NOT have a needle. But it can gently insert the friendly bacteria directly into the colon. From there, the colon knows what to do.

Using a syringe is better than using an enema because using a syringe prevents air from entering the colon. This helps in keeping the solution with friendly bacteria in the colon for a long time. A clean colon creates the best condition for the fast multiplication of friendly bacteria.

Technique of Re-Colonizing Friendly Bacteria

The procedure is to be performed before you go to bed.
1. In a cup pour 2 oz. clean, purified water.
2. Open 1-2 capsules of friendly bacteria and empty them into the water.

3. Stir.
4. You may also add 1-2 tsp. Of wheat grass juice or chlorophyl.
5. Be sure plunger of syringe is fully depressed to remove all air from syringe.
6. Submerge tip of syringe in solution.
7. Draw plunger back to fill syringe.
8. Lubricate the tip of the syringe with petroleum jelly or preferably with oil.
9. Lie down on your left side and gently insert syringe in rectum.
10. Push in plunger slowly to release the solution.
11. Remove syringe gently, wrap it in a paper towel, and let it remain in a safe place nearby, to be cleaned in the morning.

Repeat this procedure 3-7 days in a row and then 1-2 times per week during 3 or more months.

Therapeutic Effect of the Procedure

- The Small Intestine Cleansing practically cleans your whole digestive system from toxins and parasites.
- The liquid used for the procedure has a high concentration of minerals, and it works like a magnet.
- It pulls toxins from the tissues (which have less concentration of minerals) through the digestive walls and eliminates them with the feces.
- By cleansing tissues in your body you are really cleansing cells.

- This procedure will help to relax tensions and release negative emotions that are also stored in this vital organ.
- Small Intestine Cleansing cleans the digestive buds, which helps to improve the absorption of nutrients and increases digestion.
- Small Intestine Cleansing activates and improves the function of the pancreas and liver, and opens the way for direct cleansing of these vital organs.
- If you suffer from constipation, 3-5 Small Intestine Cleansings will help you overcome this problem.
- A series of these cleansings will dramatically increase your energy.
- Together with Colon Cleansings, the Small Intestine Cleansing improves the form or shape of your abdomen This because a colon and small intestine which are packed full of feces will push out your abdomen to look enlarged and unattractive.
- After the cleansing of both your colon and your small intestine, your abdomen will have a more attractive appearance and give you a thinner look.

Some Disorders and Illnesses Which Could Be Solved with Small Intestine Cleansing

Indigestion, gas, bloating, parasites, constipation, negative emotions, skin disorders, chronic fatigue, sinus problems, pancreas disorders, diabetes, ...

Self- Testing
During the Complete Small Intestine Cleansing

If you have completed 3-5 Whole Digestive System cleanses, you have removed lots of waste from your stomach, small intestine and colon. However, it doesn't mean that your digestive system doesn't have any more toxicity. You will still see much more of it releasing during this procedure. The goal of the Complete Small Intestine Cleansing is not only to remove the remaining waste from your digestive system, but also to cleanse the walls of all digestive organs and glands from toxic mucus, bile and other wastes, especially stuck to the walls of the small intestine. Small Intestine is the organ responsible for absorption of nutrients into the bloodstream. On the condition of your small intestine depends if your blood and organs contain all the necessary nutrients for their proper functioning. If your body is deprived of nutrients, your immune system weakens and health problems begin.

So what is on the walls of your Small Intestine if it has never been cleansed before?

First of all, there is toxic, sticky mucus and bile which block the digestive glands, not allowing them to produce enough digestive juices to process and break down food into nutrients and absorb them into the bloodstream. Sometimes that toxic layer forms the hard film which makes it difficult for digestive juices and nutrients to go through.

Parasites

An enormous army of parasites, bacteria, yeast and fungus occupy the small intestine. They eat the majority of nutrients, stealing them from your body. During your Small Intestine cleansing procedure you may see black, bad smelling waste and flakes, which have accumulated on the walls of your small intestine during your life, releasing through your bowels. Since this procedure cleanses not only the small intestine, but also your whole digestive system, the elimination greatly increases in volume. After the majority of waste and parasites are eliminated, cleansing of the walls and glands will begin. Pay attention to the color and consistency of the liquid you are releasing in the restroom. Sometimes the releasing liquid feels very hot. That is a reaction between minerals (you are drinking) and poisonous toxins in your intestines. Because of that, the releasing liquid is also accompanied by gas.

If you see many bubbles in the toilet, it is a sign of yeast overgrowth present in your system. Presence of yeast and other parasites make you crave sweets, carbs, chocolate, ice cream and other "junk foods". It is not surprising, because this type of food is a great nutrition for their support and reproduction, but is very harmful for humans. After you kill and flush out all parasites from your body, you would be able to control your bad cravings much easier or have none at all.

When all the "dirt" is flushed out and the liquid you are releasing is lighter, you may see it becoming a yellowish color. This is the color of toxic bile and mucus covering the walls of your small intestine. That toxic bile and mucus not only cover the walls of the small intestine, but also penetrate deep into the walls, which makes it more difficult to flush them out. Continue drinking your solution, doing light exercise and movement, and going to the restroom, until the color of release becomes the color of the solution you drink or even clear water without any particles. However, if you are physically weak or tired, during your first small intestine cleansing procedure (or sometime even second), it is not a must to get to the clear liquid. In that case you will be able to completely cleanse the walls of your digestive system and digestive glands later during following procedures, when your toxicity level lowers and your energy increases. This amazing procedure increases your energy tremendously.

Another advantage of Complete Small Intestine Cleansing

Besides cleansing of the whole digestive system and digestive glands, it works as a magnet, attracting toxins from other organs. It happens as a result of your digestive system becoming completely clean and empty after this powerful cleanse, with zero pressure inside. So the pressure in other organs and body parts is now much higher than in your digestive system and the toxicity from all other organs is being attracted to the digestive system because of the pressure difference and the magnetic powers of the solution. This "attraction" process may continue for three to five days. In order to let this process continue, you have to follow all of our dieting recommendations for those days (see the book *"Eight Steps to Perfect Health"* cleansing the small intestine chapter).

When toxic elements from other organs reach the digestive system, they accumulate in the large intestine and from there are flushed out by the follow up Colon cleansing procedure 2-4 days after your Complete Small Intestine

Cleansing. During the follow up Colonic, you will also partially cleanse liver, pancreas, sinuses, lungs and other vital organs. Complete cleansing of your whole digestive system removes the main blood poisoning source. Now, if you start eating right and your digestive system is free of toxicity, your blood is not being fed by new "dirt". To fully cleanse your blood vessels and remove toxins already present in your bloodstream, it is important to completely cleanse the Liver–the main blood filter, and do juice therapy according to the developed program by our center.

SELF HELP:　　　*LIVER AND DIGESTION*

Recipe to strengthen the digestion and activation of the liver. Shred 3 medium beets and put in a 3 quart glass jar. Add: handful of raisins, a whole garlic (peeled), 1 cup of sugar. Cover with 2.5 qts. Room temperature water. Mix well together and add a small piece of black bread. Cover the jar with cheesecloth and store in a dark place for three days. Once the beverage is ready, drink 4-6 oz before meals. To make sure that the beverage does not spoil, strain it 5 days later and put in the refrigerator. Before drinking, warmup to room temperature.

Step #4

Complex Liver Cleansing

"Helping your major blood filter to normalize cholesterol."

The Liver: Your First Line of Defense Against Disease

The liver is the most important organ in the entire human immune system because its primary function is to remove harmful chemicals and unwelcome microscopic organisms that cause disease.

Sources of chemical and biological toxins are numerous in our environment, and include automobile and truck exhaust, preservatives commonly used in processed foods, nicotine, chemical fumes from manufactured products, airborne dust and microbes, pharmaceuticals and other drugs, alcohol, fats in foods, and poorly cleaned foods. As these toxins enter the human body, they will slowly poison your health unless removed.

The way the liver removes these contaminants is by filtering them from the blood stream, and then sending these poisonous wastes to the excretory organs. As it goes about the business of filtering, the liver too often experiences the very same problem all filters have: It becomes clogged with the material which it is filtering. This leads to three problems.

First, the contaminants clogging the liver are literally stored in this organ instead of being transported for removal via urination or defecation. As these unwelcome chemicals and microscopic organisms accumulate and concentrate over time, the liver is slowly poisoned by them.

Second, toxins stored in the liver build up in size over time and create very real physical pressure inside the liver. This physical pressure interferes with the ability of fluids to flow freely within the liver. It impairs the blood's access to the filtering work of the liver.

Third, because these contaminants clog the liver, its ability to filter out new contaminants is lessened. The amount of this decrease in function is proportional to the amount of filter pores which are clogged. Since the liver is not able to filter at maximum efficiency, toxins are not being removed from the blood stream. This means more chemical and biological toxins are circulated to all of the organs and tissues in the body. These toxins are stored at the cellular level and slowly poison those organs and tissues.

The bottom line is that a liver bloated with masses of chemical and biological toxins is not only less able to fight simple sicknesses such as colds and flu, but is weakened in the fight against the more serious diseases such as cancer, etc.

Add to this the toxins building up in the rest of your body and you get poor health generally, and an increased vulnerability to the diseases to which you are genetically prone. Since **the liver is the power player in the immune**

system, you cannot afford to have your star athlete in the game of good health to be on the bench or on the way to the hospital because modern contaminants have begun to choke the life out of it.

The famous Indian doctor Shevananda said that about 90% of health disorders come from a weakened liver. The latest medical research shows that all degenerative diseases (cancer, arthritis, diabetes, asthma, etc.) are created by the dysfunction of a liver which is blocked and overloaded with toxic waste material.

Side Effects of Having a Toxic Liver

The liver performs other critical functions. It participates in digestion, metabolism, and the proper working of the gall bladder.

The gall bladder and the liver work in close harmony as well as close proximity. Accumulated toxins in the liver slow down the secretion of bile from the gall bladder. This results in bile crystallization and the formation of gall bladder stones.

Although the liver is the key organ in the immune system, the lymphatic system, the circulatory system, the spleen, and the bone marrow are also part of the immune system. The stronger each individual member of the immune system is, the better they work together and the stronger the entire immune system is.

An unclean liver means unclean blood which blocks the tiny ducts in the thyroid gland.

The Good News

Fortunately, the health-robbing toxic wastes stored in the liver can be removed naturally under the guidance of a trained professional. Using techniques developed and enhanced over the centuries, the human liver can be coaxed into gently releasing, not only the original contaminants entering the body, but also their by-products such as cholesterol, fat, pathologic mucous, stagnated bile, and bilirubin stones.

Since "an ounce of prevention is worth a pound of cure," a liver cleansing will allow you to take powerful steps towards fighting off life-threatening disease, debilitating illnesses, and common sicknesses. It will help you to feel healthier and enjoy life more since the nasty toxins that once choked your liver are gone.

Nine-Organ Cleansing Procedure

Liver cleansing in our Center is a complex cleansing of nine important body organs: **stomach, pancreas, liver, gall bladder, spleen, small intestine, colon, blood, and thyroid gland.**

Benefits of a Complex Liver Cleansing

- Enhanced ability to clean the bloodstream.
- Stronger immune system.
- Loss of toxic waste and weight.
- Improved metabolism.
- Cleaner skin.
- Improved digestion.

- Greater protection from degenerative diseases such as cancer, arthritis, diabetes, and asthma.

Additional Benefits of Complex Liver Cleansing

A full Complex Liver Cleansing automatically cleanses the gall bladder, the pancreatic gland, and the spleen. It also helps cleanse the small intestine and the colon while strengthening the lymphatic and circulatory systems. Additionally, proper liver cleansing improves the tone of the kidneys and the thyroid gland. Clean blood helps to cleanse the thyroid gland and improve its function.

Because the liver is naturally divided into four parts, or quadrants, and since each cleansing will cleanse only one part, **full Complex Liver Cleansing requires four separate procedures.**

During Complex Liver Cleansing, toxic wastes released by the above organs go first into the small intestine then on to the colon. These wastes are then best removed by Colon Cleansing that gently flushes these toxic wastes out of the body before they can adhere to the colon walls.

SELF HELP: *GALLBLADDER STONES*

If your doctor diagnosed you with gallbladder stones: Wash thoroughly 2 lbs of potatoes (not peeled) and cover with 3 qts of water. Boil until half of the liquid is left. Mash the potatoes and leave over night. In the morning, drain the liquid and drink 4 oz before meals 1-2 weeks before your liver cleansing procedure.

Instructions
for Complex
Liver Cleansing

Our Complex Liver Cleansing is different from liver cleansings described in other books.

The first disadvantage of other liver cleansings is that you do not have a fully trained health professional—with experience in liver cleansing—to personally tailor the procedure to your particular circumstances.

Second, you have no professional guidance during the procedure, or anyone of whom to ask questions as they arise.

The third disadvantage is the lack of preparation. When one properly prepares for this (or any) cleansing procedure, the procedure is more effective. This is often because the toxic masses and stones (gall stones and liver stones) are softened by proper preparation, and therefore exit more fully from the organ being cleansed. **Without this preparation** the desired results are decreased, and you may feel really bad during the cleansing.

The fourth disadvantage is that most liver cleansings do not call for the small intestine to be cleansed prior to the liver cleansing. This is important because the small intestine is the organ into which the liver discards its toxins during the liver cleansing. If the small intestine is blocked with accumulated wastes, the movement of the newly released liver toxins is slowed. When these wastes are slowed down in the small intestine and the colon there is a greater chance for them to stick to the walls of these two organs, and a greater chance that the wastes will be reabsorbed.

Preparing the Body for Complex Liver Cleansing

In our Center, we do much preparation before Complex Liver Cleansing. We carefully cleanse the whole digestive system to assist in the removal of toxic bile and other liver wastes (as described above). In addition, we use juice therapy, Far Infrared Radiation (FIR), massage of internal organs, reflexology, and infrared sauna to soften accumulated wastes.

Complex Liver Cleansing is the best beginning for Cell Cleansing. The combination of these two cleansings is a powerful way to help to heal many diseases, rejuvenate the body, and lose toxic weight.

ATTENTION: *Read and understand this material very carefully.*

Preparation for Complex Liver Cleansing

1. *Do a Series of 2-3 Colon Cleansings, About 2 Whole Digestive System Cleansings, and 1-2 Small Intestine Cleansings before the Complex Liver Cleansing.* This is necessary because accumulated toxic waste materials from the liver go through the small intestines and the colon, as described above.

2. One or two weeks before the Complex Liver Cleansing, start to take a warm bath two or three times a week. Don't stay in the bath more than 15 to 20 minutes. Two to three cups of sea salt or Epsom salt can be added to the bath. A warm bath helps to soften up the toxicity and facilitates its removal.

3. Switch to the vegetarian diet for three to seven days before Complex Liver Cleansing. This gives the liver an opportunity to accumulate strength and energy to expel the toxins.

4. Those with serious illnesses or excess weight should go on juice therapy (juice fasting) for **three days** right before Complex Liver Cleansing. (To lose more weight you may fast for four days). Those who are weak or afraid of losing any weight may go on juice therapy for one day right before Complex Liver Cleansing. During these days you may drink distilled water and juices freshly made if possible. During the first two days, drink carrot, carrot-apple, and apple juices at your own discretion. On the third day it is better to drink apple juice only, or the juice of 4-5 apples plus one lemon. Drink one or two glasses approximately every two hours. If possible, use only organic carrots. When choosing the variety of apple, it is preferable to buy "Granny Smith." Juices absorb into the bloodstream, go through the liver, flush it, and activate the flow of stagnated bile. **If you have problems with yeast,** drink 1 cup of juice followed by 1 cup of water or dandelion root tea to dilute the concentration of sugar. If the yeast problem is severe,

you may drink water with lemon instead of apple juice.

5. On the third day of juice therapy, you will receive a colon cleansing with FIR. You also have an option to add a highly recommended gall bladder / liver massage, a foot reflexology massage, and infrared sauna that day (some programs already include these procedures). To understand FIR, see my book, *Deep Internal Body Cleansing,* chapter entitled, Heavy Metal Cleansing and the FIR Sauna chapter in this book.

These procedures activate the liver, expand its ducts, and prepare the way for the passage of toxins.

The concluding part of the procedure is performed by the client at home after receiving detailed instructions. (See below.) At this time you will pick up from the Center the solution for Complex Liver Cleansing for consumption at home.

*If you suffer from illnesses related to liver functioning (cholesterol, high blood pressure, allergies, etc), in addition to the cleansing procedures, regularly drink fresh beet/apple juice. Also apply light heat to the liver (heating pad or warm bath) for 15 min. twice/ day.

The First Day of Complex Liver Cleansing

The first day of Complex Liver Cleansing is the same as the third day of juice therapy (as described above).

This first day is divided into two parts: (a) procedures performed in the Center, and (b) procedures performed at home. (For procedures performed at the Center see #5 above.)

76

Once you have completed the procedures to be performed in the Center on this first day you will go home with the carefully prepared, organic solution for oral consumption.

At approximately **7:00 p.m.** begin the procedures described below. (This assumes that you normally keep waking hours that most people keep.) The reason for this timing is that the procedures you will perform at home cause the majority of toxins to exit the liver between 1and 3 a.m. This is the biorhythmic time when the liver is most active. You should be finished with the procedures below in about four hours. * *The earlier you begin, the more energy your system will have to release toxins.*

Sequence of Steps:

Notice: Two hours before drinking Solution #1, do not drink anything, including water.

-Prepare your bed
-Put (warmed) solution near your bed.
-Prepare chopped garlic in a closed container.
-Prepare a piece of lemon on a plate near your bed.
-Prepare a piece of pickle or ginger on a plate near your bed.
-Have a timer near your bed.

1. Take a **warm** bath for 15 to 20 minutes. The bath doesn't have to be very hot, but the hotter you can tolerate it the better. At the end of your bath, and before you stand up, flush your face and forehead with cool water. When you stand up from the bath do so very slowly. These precautions are necessary for people with weak vessels and unstable blood pressure, to avoid dizziness and falling. Be careful!

2.	From the bath go directly to the bed, couch, or comfy arm chair. Lie down on your right side (where the liver is) with your head and chest elevated so as to create better drainage. Put a warm heating pad or water bottle under your right side (on the liver area). **IT IS VERY IMPORTANT THAT YOU NEVER FALL ASLEEP ON A HEATING PAD. YOU CAN GET BURNED IN THIS FASHION.** This is another reason for having a timer next to the bed, just in case you fall asleep on the bed. If the heating pad or water bottle is too hot for you, cover it with a towel. Make sure you feel no tightness or contraction in the liver area.

3.	Warm the solution provided by the Center in a double boiler pan to body temperature before going to bath, or have someone warm it for you during your bath. If you have a problem drinking it warm, drink it at room temperature. After lying down on your right side with a heating pad or water bottle, raise your body on your elbow and . . .

*a.	Drink solution #1.*

You will notice that the solution is a two-phase liquid. It is recommended that you **do not to try to mix the solution.** It is also recommended that you drink the solution with moderate speed without stopping. After you drink the solution, lie down on the heating pad/hot water bottle on your right side immediately. Rest for 15 minutes.

b.   ***Drink solution #2.***   Rest 20 minutes.

c.   ***Drink solution #3.***   Rest 20 minutes.

d.   ***Drink solution #4.***   Rest 25 minutes.

e.   ***Drink solution #5.***   Rest 25 to 30 minutes

f.   ***Drink solution #6.*** (If you are small, the first time you will receive 5 jars instead of 6. If your weight is more than 200 pounds, on the second Liver Cleanse you may receive more than 6 jars.)

* To help your liver, gallbladder, pancreas and spleen release toxins better, after each container that you drink, perform 3-5 abdominal and rib breathing exercises described in my book "Healing Through Cleansing 3".

Continue lying on your right side for one more hour after you finish drinking the solution. If lying on the right side becomes difficult, it is permitted periodically (for one or two minutes) to turn on your back.

After one hour, it is okay to lie on your back and on your right side. Try not to lie on the left side or on the abdomen.

Everybody is different. If you find it uncomfortable to lie down, you are allowed to sit in a comfortable chair with the heating pad tied snugly around you while drinking your solution. One to one-and-one-half (1-1½) hours after drinking your solution, you may lie in bed on your right side or on your back.

The drinking solution contains a large amount of oil so there will be a strong impulse from the liver and gall bladder to push out bile to break down the fat. Because the small intestine is empty with the duct open, and the liver contents are softened by juice, it will be able to push out a large amount of toxins like cholesterol, chemicals, medicines, stones and stagnant bile along with the new bile.

From the small intestine, the toxins go to the large intestine and then to the exit. Sometimes, it is possible to hear "the breathing" of the liver, that is, movement of the stones, mucous, stagnated bile, and other toxins.

Some people, as the result of incorrect and excessive food intake, might have a half-open position of the valve between the stomach and small intestines. In this case, dissolved toxic bile, mucous, and other toxic components of the liver which are dissolved because of the drinking solution, and also some of the solution itself, might come through into the stomach and create nausea. This is not unusual.

During light nausea there are some things you can do to help. Find the one that works best for you:

1. Open the container with cut garlic and inhale the vapor from it.
2. Gargle with freshly made lemon juice, or suck a piece of lemon (don't eat it).
3. Put a piece of pickle or ginger in the mouth and suck the juice from it. DO NOT EAT IT.
4. Press on the point of your face, right under your nose and right over your upper lip. Press it for 10 to 15 seconds. Do not press too hard.

If nausea becomes stronger and the above methods don't help, try to tolerate it for two or three hours after drinking the last jar of solution. During this time try to relax and rest; try not to move, or to move as little as possible.

Then, if the nausea has not gone away, try to induce vomiting by stimulating the root of the tongue with two fingers. Do it several times, until your stomach is empty. If vomiting does not happen, drink 1-2 cups of very warm water and repeat stimulation of the root of the tongue. The water will help and make it easier for you to cleanse your stomach. After that, flush your mouth with cool, clean water.

Although it is preferable to have the wastes from the liver exit via the colon, if the body calls for you to vomit this material it is better to do so. You will thank yourself afterward, because you will feel better immediately.

Lie down, relax, and rest. If possible, ask your relatives to massage your feet. Then put a warm water bottle to your feet.

After vomiting, you may experience a burning sensation in your stomach and in your mouth. It is normal and will go away. It happens because of the toxic bile and other materials from the liver.

Thirty minutes to one hour after vomiting, or four hours after drinking the last jar of solution, you may drink hot herbal tea from camomile and peppermint, with honey, which will decrease or even eliminate any unpleasant tastes.

Regardless of the unpleasantness of vomiting, it does have its positive side. It graphically demonstrates what the liver has had to put up with "for all these years."

Vomiting also helps to clean and activate the pancreatic gland, and to clean the bottom of the stomach from stagnated bile and other toxins. It also helps to improve digestion and improves the work of the valve between the stomach and small intestine.

The Second Day of Complex Liver Cleansing

Depending on your condition, you may be advised to have a Small Intestine Cleansing or Whole Digestive System Cleansing, and in some cases a Colon Cleansing

In the morning, after waking up, take a warm shower and clean your teeth, mouth and tongue. Then you may drink one glass of warm water with lemon juice or apple cider vinegar (1 tsp. to 8 oz.), or hot herbal tea (no sweeteners). Do not eat any food before the Whole Digestive System Cleansing or the Small Intestine Cleansing. If you are doing a Colon Cleansing, and if you do not feel nauseous, you may drink carrot or apple juice plus beet juice, 1-2 cups.

Do a few gymnastic exercises and light walking.

If you have bowel movements, pay attention to what comes out. You may observe dark green or light green liver stones up to one-half inch in length. These liver stones can assume a variety of shapes, from football to irregular to amorphous. What you are seeing is toxic mucous, toxic bile, excess cholesterol, the residue of alcoholic beverages, drugs (prescription or other), and various other wastes. These stones are accumulated with help of parasites. It is them, "architects" and "builders" who create these stones. They pick up bile, cholesterol, mucus and build their homes in the form of a stone. Thousands of colonies of parasites/infection is in each stone. These parasites produce poisons, lay eggs and damage healthy cells of the liver, disturbing it's function. These wastes have a very unpleasant smell. Just remember that you never have to be afflicted with this toxic waste again. It is gone.

Some people are slower to eject toxins from the liver, and some people's systems are slower to move these toxins through the intestinal tract. In this case, you will see toxins from the liver only during the procedure at the office.

The second day must be your day off from work both in the office and at home. Your body has just expended a lot of energy to get rid of decades of toxins so it is normal for you to feel weak. This weakness will be offset by the strength you will begin to gather from having a rejuvenated liver and other organs. Whatever weakness, nausea, and other unpleasant sensations you may experience will go away quickly.

On the second day of Complex Liver Cleansing, you may receive some of the following cleansing procedures:
1.   Stomach Cleansing.
2.   Colon Cleansing.
3.   Small Intestine Cleansing.
4.   Sinus Cleansing.
5.   Sauna.
6.   Full Body Cleansing Massage.

The most important procedure following a Liver Cleanse is Colon Cleansing. Other procedures add benefits and increase the amount of toxins eliminated from the liver and other organs and prevent re-absorption.

30 minutes to 1 hour after colon hydrotherapy, you may eat cooked brown rice with Ghee.

Some Other Useful Advice

1.   Try to follow the instructions to the letter. Any changes must be reconciled. Violating instructions

will decrease the benefits of the cleansing or may even harm you.

2. During this cleansing, it is not recommended to take any drugs. If you have to take pharmaceuticals, let us know about them before cleansing.

3. Do not combine Complex Liver Cleansing with a dental appointment or with anesthesia. If you need to see a dentist, do it before Complex Liver Cleansing.

4. Do no get upset if during the Complex Liver Cleansing you do not see any stones. Everything you eliminate during the Complex Liver Cleansing (stones, toxic bile, mucus, etc.) is poison and its elimination improves your health. Sometimes good preparation and juices dilute liver and gall bladder stones and transform them to green black, sticky liquid.

First Week after Complex Liver Cleansing

After the procedure of Complex Liver Cleansing, the liver will stay open and continue ejection of toxins for five to seven days. Some of these toxins will be collecting in the large intestine, so it is recommended to do another Colon Cleansing in 3-5 days after Complex Liver Cleansing.

During this time, you should not overeat or choose gas producing foods such as beans. Gas expands your stomach and creates pressure on the liver. This stops this process of continuing to eliminate toxins. During these days, the diet must be vegetarian.

You will be surprised to see the toxins coming out. However, if during that time, you have a blood, urine, saliva, or any other test done, it will show a high level of toxicity. If you plan to have any test after the Liver Cleanse, wait for at least two weeks, so you can have the real picture of what is happening in your body.

Many people have a burst of energy 1-3 days after the procedure and try to catchup on everything they haven't done in months. Then the following day and for days after, they may feel very tired and exhausted. If you do receive that great gifs of energy, please enjoy it. Just stay relaxed, take a nice walk or do some light work. Give a chance for that energy to heal your mind, body and soul.

Therapeutic Benefits

Benefits derived from a Complex Liver Cleansing are priceless. These include:
- Strengthened immune system.
- Increased energy level.
- Greater sense of well-being.

You will be able to feel this condition only when your liver is completely clean. For this reason, it is necessary to keep on cleansing it until ejection stops.

In the first year, it is recommended to do five to seven Complex Liver Cleansings. The frequency of the procedure depends on individual tolerance.

Then for liver support, one Complex Liver Cleansing per year is enough.

Some Disorders and Illnesses Which Could Be Solved with Complex Liver Cleansing

Gall stones, high cholesterol, allergies, skin problems, digestive problems, hepatitis, thyroid disorders, constipation, headaches, parasites, anger, insomnia, ...

Self-Testing
During the
Complex Liver Cleansing

You may begin self-testing even during your preparation (juice fast) for the actual liver cleansing procedure.

Things to look for

If during your juice fast you have a headache or weakness it is a signal of high toxicity in your stomach. You may immediately have a question-- where did that stomach toxicity come from, if I already cleansed my stomach so many times? Some clients' stomachs are so clogged and covered with toxicity, that even after a few cleanses, parts of that toxicity is still there. Sometimes toxins from other organs especially from lungs and sinuses are also being released in your stomach. **To lower or neutralize the toxicity level in your stomach, you may do the following...**

Take a glass of purified water (8oz) and add two teaspoons of Organic Apple Cider Vinegar (you can buy it in any Health Food Store). Sit as still as possible and drink that cocktail two sips every 5 minutes until the headache is gone. If one glass is not enough, you may drink two or even three glasses. This technique will definitely help if your headache is caused by toxicity. You may also put your feet in the washbowl with hot water for 10-15 minutes. When the water starts cooling off, you have to keep adding hot water to maintain the temperature. Hot water will pul the blood from your head down to your feet and lower the blood pressure in the head and also remove part of toxicity through the open pores of your feet. It should make you feel much better.

If during your preparation fasting you experience too much gas and discomfort in your abdomen, it usually indicates that you drink your juice too fast, like water, not holding every sip in your mouth to mix it with saliva. It creates indigestion and accumulation of excess gasses which put pressure on the walls of your digestive organs and create discomfort, pain and fatigue. In order to prevent these problems, it is necessary to hold each sip in your mouth for 10-20 seconds or more. Drinking hot water with lemon between your juices is also helpful.

If while fasting you feel hunger, it means you are not drinking enough juice. On the other hand, if you drink too much juice, you may experience light nausea, fatigue or even a "sugar-rush". So it is a must to alternate juice with water or hot tea (preferably dandelion root tea). Make sure that the temperature of water is not too hot, it should not burn your lips.

During your Liver Cleanse

If during or after drinking your liver solution you feel nausea or fatigue, it indicates clogginess of your stomach walls with toxicity or improper functioning of the valve located between the stomach and the small intestine. In it's normal state, the valve should be closed and open only after the food has been processed by digestive juices, then the valve allows it to go down to the small intestine. Wrong food combining, overeating and eating late results in the malfunctioning of the valve and it stays slightly open at all times, allowing the food just slide into your small intestine before it is completely processed creating excess gas and toxicity. On the other hand, bile produced to digest fats in the small intestine, is able to get into the stomach through the open valve, causing acid reflex, heartburn, headache, nausea and other problems. So this way during your liver cleansing procedure, toxicity from your liver can also get into your stomach through the open valve and create fatigue and nausea.

If nausea increases, wait 2-3 hours after the intake of the last liver solution, then put two fingers in your mouth and press on the root of your tongue to induce vomiting. It would help to drink a cup or two of warm, lightly salted water first to make it easier and less straining. Even though it seems very unpleasant, by vomiting, you will cleanse your stomach walls, close the valve and improve your digestion and quickly make you feel better.

If that same night, after drinking the liver solution you are not able to have a bowel movement on your own it indicates weakness of your digestive system. In order to improve function of your digestive system, it is necessary to cleanse the liver completely by repeating it 4-5 times. It is also important to maintain the health of your liver by repeating Liver cleansing 1-2 times per year in fall and spring.

What comes out of you during the liver cleanse?

Ideally, in order to see what exactly your Liver is releasing, it is best to have your bowel movement not into the toilet, but into the medium size bowl. The toilet is always full of water, so you won't see an exact picture.

Plus, the water will dilute the color, consistency and smell of reality. This way you get wrong perception and think that you have released very little and can't even feel the toxic poisonous smell. So to see the real picture, get a small or medium bowl and if you feel an urge to eliminate at night or the next morning of your cleanse, use the bowl instead of the toilet. This is a better way to see what you are carrying in your liver–the chemical lab of your body, which is designed to cleanse your blood and protect you from illnesses. When you see how much "dirt" you have in your liver, you may finally understand where all your health problems are coming from.

There is another way to see what you are releasing during the Liver cleansing procedure. Get a large pasta strainer and put it over the toilet-bowl when you have your elimination. Liquid substances will go through, but the stones will stay in the strainer. If the stones are covered in fecal color, you may wash them off with water. The fecal cover will come off and you will see dark and light green stones from your gallbladder and liver. You may also use the strainer for few more days, even after you start eating. During that time, liver is still releasing toxins, which of course mix with regular bowel and you are not able to see anything. If you use the strainer, you may wash off the regular fecal matter with water and see undissolved liver/gallbladder stones. By using this technique, you may see for yourself that the toxic elimination from the liver continues for 5-7 days. In order not to stop that process, we recommend to follow our strict dieting recommendations for that time (See book *"Eight Steps to perfect Health"*) and also have a follow up colonic 2-4 days later.

What exactly do you see?

Please understand that whatever you release during your liver cleanse is not just regular intestinal waste. All the cleanses you had done prior to it; fasting and cleansing procedures before your liver cleanse removed everything from your digestive system. So everything you see during your liver cleansing procedure (liquid and solid) comes from the liver, gallbladder and pancreas.

The stones you see, may be different sizes from tiny to large, from just a few to hundreds. Sometimes, the juices you drink and heat (from FIR, baths or heating pad) dissolve stones into gooey substance. It does not indicate unsuccessful cleanse, on the contrary, it means that you prepared very well. Whatever comes out of you during the Liver cleansing in any form, liquid or solid, consists of cholesterol, alcohol, chemicals from food, medication, dead cells, inorganic minerals, parasites, bilirubin, toxic mucus and bile, etc.

Toxic mucus is a result of mucus forming foods, such as bread, pasta, cheese and other dairy products, ice cream and other sweets. Toxic bile is a result of late meals, overeating, excess amounts of proteins and fats.

You may also notice tiny stones or sand released from the pancreas. Pancreas of a modern person with "normal" eating habits is 2-4 times larger than it should be. It is full with sand and mucus, and is not able to perform its normal functions. Pancreas is a very important gland responsible for the sugar level in the blood as well as it helps the liver to dissolve fats.

Why you can not have a liver cleanse without proper preparation?

Digestive system holds a great amount of toxicity, which on one hand blocks the pathway for liver toxicity to be eliminated, and on the other hand elimination of liver toxicity and all digestive toxins at once is too overwhelming and shocking for the system. For that reason we use a gentle and safe technique of proper preparation. First, we cleanse your digestive system and open the pathway for liver toxicity. Only than, when all the pathways are open, you may have an actual Liver cleansing procedure. If done in that order, more toxicity from the liver will be removed, it will not get stuck on its way and the effect will be much higher leaving you feeling much better afterward.

Everything you release from the liver, gallbladder and pancreas, no matter what it looks like or how much comes out, plays a tremendous role in improving your health; prevention; fighting and winning over illnesses and parasites. Every Liver cleansing procedure you do, is a celebration for your body, strengthening your health and prolonging your life.

Note: *The described above liver cleansing method is the base method used in our center. However, some programs, depending on clients' individuality and financial circumstances, number of cleansing procedures included in the complex liver cleansing might vary. However, the main principal- detailed preparation for the procedure, complete or partial cleansing of the digestive system second day after the procedure, as well as the colon cleansing 3-7 days after liver cleansing– stays the same and unchanged.*

Step #5

Joint Cleansing

"Removing joint pain
and increasing
flexibility."

Cleansing the Joints, Spine and Tissues

The pathway to preventing joint pain, and even to
lessening its painful effects for those who already have joint
pain, is found first in understanding its causes and then in
cleansing the body of those causes.

The Cause of It All

It is no surprise to those who suffer from joint pains,
such as arthritis, that the pointed stabbing sensation in those
aching joints comes from the formation of needle-shaped
crystals. These crystals are created from uric acid, a
substance found in animal proteins. The typical American
eats much more meat than people in other cultures, and
consequently we have a high incidence of arthritis in this
country.

Diet is not the only thing that can lead to the formation of uric acid crystals. Heredity and a lack of physical activity play a part as well. Organs that have never been cleansed can tend to create conditions favorable to uric acid formation.

Despite all of this, the prudent person can use his or her mind to prevent joint pain caused by such dietary contamination. Indeed, if the physical condition of the afflicted joints is not too far advanced, it may be possible to decrease the pain or in some cases even eliminate the pain.

Why and How It Hurts?

Most uric acid crystals form in joints, including the spinal column around the disks. These crystals are hard enough to cause actual wear and tear to these bones.

Unfortunately, other things also can cause physical injury to the joints and the spine: being overweight, lifting very heavy items, very sharp injuring movements and direct blows to the joints. An insufficient amount of sinovial fluid, which acts as a lubricant for the joints, can also lead to bone wear and tear.

One of the many disadvantages that comes from uric acid crystals is that they put pressure on veins and energy channels making blood and energy circulation slower. This can cause the limbs to get cold more easily, leading to extra stiffness in the joints.

Bony materials are not the only part of the body to suffer from the formation of uric acid crystals. These unwelcome mineral needles can form in soft tissue as well, such as the upper-back/shoulders zone. When they do, they tend to scratch the tissues. The reason for uric acid crystals being formed in soft tissues is usually poor blood circulation. This, in turn, is sometimes the result of sitting in an uncomfortable position for too long, and by stress. With time, if no corrective measures are taken, discomfort and pain can occur and increase in the area of shoulders and neck.

All of these situations and conditions can add together to bring unremitting pain to some people. The goal of Koyfman Whole Body Cleansing is to use natural healing techniques to remove one of the greatest causes of joint and spine pain, the uric acid crystals.

Bringing Relief

Employing natural healing techniques developed over the centuries, and using state-of-the-art equipment Koyfman Whole Body Cleansing dissolves the uric acid crystals, causing them to be washed easily out of the joints, spine and tissues. The liquefied uric acid is then transported by the circulatory system from the joints, spine and tissues to the waste elimination organs of the body. There is no other way to remove this source of pain, not even surgery.

If you have a serious problem with your joints because of the accumulation of uric acid crystals, then this cleansing must be repeated four or five times during the first year. Then, depending on your personal circumstances and your lifestyle and dietary choices, Joint Cleansing can be continued one or two times a year.

Therapeutic Effects of Joint Cleansing

- Removes certain unhealthy chemicals from your body, naturally and gently.
- May lessen or eliminate pain in areas affected by uric acid crystals.
- May prevent the onset of illnesses caused by uric acid.
- May increase the flexibility and range of motion in joints and/or the spine.
- May make everyday movement easier and exercise better or possible.
- May increase the blood flow in joints, spine and tissues.
- May increase mental concentration since pain is no longer distracting you.
- May make you less vulnerable to changes in the weather.
- May increase physical energy

The specific benefits that each person experiences depends on many interrelated factors, including your own personal body chemistry, the extent of uric acid development, and your diet and exercise. One thing is undisputed: The gentle, natural removal of uric acid is beneficial to your health, especially to the joints.

Instructions
for
Joint Cleansing

The Causes

What causes a sharp increased pains which sometimes are felt by those suffering from uric acid crystals?

1. Physical fatigue.
2. Pollution of the large intestine.
3. Poor kidney function.
4. The common cold.
5. Negative energy coming from humidity inside buildings, extra moisture from long rains, etc.
6. Long time spent in places where natural magnetic lines intersect, exposure to powerful electromagnetic vibrations (proximity to electric plants) and underground anomalies (underground water, accumulated metals, alloys, vacuums).
7. Frequent emotional stresses.
8. Not enough water.
9. Use of alcohol and overuse of salt in food.
10. Parasites.

Now that we have a brief background on what causes joint, spine and tissue pain, how do we go about preventing these unwelcome needle-shaped intruders? And how do we go about lessening the joint pain some people suffer from the accumulation of uric acid crystals?

Preparation for Joint Cleansing

Before you begin the actual Joint Cleansing, it is necessary to cleanse from toxicity your whole digestive system, liver and lymph. It will strengthen you body as a whole and open all the channels of toxin excretion.

Order of cleansing procedures to prepare for Joint Cleansing

1. Cleanse the large intestine (colon) from waste, parasites, gas and excessive pressure.
2. Whole Digestive System Cleansing
3. Complete Small Intestine Cleansing
4. Complex Liver Cleansing
5. Complete Lymph Cleansing

Diet, Exercise and Heat

1. Practice a raw vegetarian diet. 15% to 20% cooked food is allowed. Organic food is preferred.
2. Maintain a program of exercises for joints and spine.
3. Engage in special mind exercises for joints daily.
4. Use dry heat (dry sauna).

Detailed Instructions for Joint Cleansing
(Diet, Juices, Herbs) Duration of cleansing: 3 weeks.

Start and maintain a vegetarian diet. If your digestion is normal, your food should be 80-85% raw. Joint cleansing is done with the help of special herbs. Because these herbs wash out, not only toxic crystals, but also minerals that are necessary for basic health, these lost, good minerals must be replaced by drinking three or four glasses of freshly made, organic juices, and liquid minerals like seasilver and noni juice. You may choose from the following combinations:

- Carrots and celery (6:2 ratio)
- Carrots, cucumber and beet (10:3:3 ratio)
- Carrots, celery and parsley (9:5:2 ratio)
- Grapefruit

These juices must be made from fresh, ripe produce. They must *never* come from a can. They must never be processed such as dried, frozen, etc.

Because the body is also losing potassium, it is necessary to eat foods which contain potassium. These include: potatoes, millet, bananas, apples, soaked raisins, dried apricots, and apple cider vinegar.

Add flaxseed oil to salads.

Raw products and juices give the body necessary minerals and vitamins; they also cool it down. To restore the heat balance one must:

1. During the day, drink 4 to 6 cups of hot herbal tea, such as rose hips, parsley, or dandelion root.
2. Every day between 5 p.m. and 9 p.m., take a hot bath with sea salt (3-4 cups of salt for one bath).
3. Daily dry brush massage for 10 minutes.

4.   Every day, 30 minutes of mind joint exercises.
5.   **Procedures in the Center:**
          Massage and Sauna, 2 or 3 times per week
          Colon Cleansing, 1 or 2 times per week

Directions for Taking the Herbal Solution

3 days of taking herbs
    7 day break
3 days of taking herbs
    7 day break
7 days of kidney cleansing

The process of dissolving the uric acid crystals and making them move from the joints, spine and tissues happens, not only during the days you take the herbs, but also during the breaks. Therefore, one must follow the program in order to make it work at maximum. Koyfman Whole Body Cleansing will provide you with packets from which you will make a special solution to enhance the cleansing. These will be taken during the three days of taking herbs.

Method of Preparing the Herbal Solution

Put one packet in a pan with 12 oz. of clean water. Heat to boiling and then let simmer for five minutes. Put this mixture in a thermos and let it stay for three hours. Then strain the solution and put in your refrigerator.

Next day start drinking one teaspoon every 15 minutes until done (6 or 8 hours).

If you miss your planned time to drink, continue with the same amount and scheduled time. Do not increase the dosage as that can be bad for your stomach.

How Does the Elimination of Toxic Crystals Occur?

Elements contained in the herbal solution and the freshly-made juices dissolve the uric acid crystals causing them to wash out easily from the joints, spine and tissues. The dissolved uric acid is then transported by the circulatory system to the kidneys and eliminated with the urine.

For those who want proof that the procedure is working, try the following experiment: Each morning collect your first urine in a clean glass jar. Then leave this urine in a cool, dark place such as a closet that is rarely opened. (Make sure children and pets will not find this collection.) After about three or four weeks kept tightly sealed in a cool, dark place, the uric acid will re-crystalize in the collected urine and precipitate to the bottom of the container. Now you can see what was in your joints, spine and tissues.

Dissolved toxins also flow to the large intestine (colon) during this procedure. This is due to the creation of a lower pressure in the colon as compared to other organs. To help this process, it is recommended that you not eat for four hours after Colon Cleansing. During that time you may drink cleansing tea and freshly-made organic juices. The next Colon Cleansing will show you again how much uric acid can be drawn from your system. You will see this in the color of the wastes.

Procedures Done at Home to Help the Joint Cleansing and Pain Relief.

The hot bath with sea salt and the dry sauna help relieve the load on your kidneys by pulling the toxins through the skin. The dry brush massage activates skin respiration and facilitates the work of the lungs to eliminate toxic gasses formed during the process of cleansing. A long walk of one or more hours activates the lungs and the elimination of toxic gasses.

Mind exercises for joints, not only activate blood flow in the joints and the spine, but also improve the flow of energy through the energy channels and the connection between the brain and the joints.

Directions for Mind Exercises for the Joints

1. Sit in a comfortable chair and close your eyes.
2. Visualize someone standing in front of you at a distance at which you can see that person clearly.
3. Who you choose to visualize is up to you. It should be someone who will not distract you from this mind exercise.
4. Visualize this person doing joint exercises beginning with toes and working all the way to the top of the head, 10 repetitions for each movement.
5. See this person lift the left leg, and curl and relax the left toes ten times.
6. See this person flex the ankle, forward and back, side to side, circular clockwise and then counterclockwise.
7. See this person stretch and bend the knee forward and back, side to side, and circular both directions.

101

8. See this person move the leg at the hip, forward and back, side to side, and circular both directions.
9. Then see this person do the same with the other leg, toes, ankle, knee, and hip.
10. See this person flex and twist the spine forward and back, sideways, and circular both ways.
11. See this person flex the fingers, wrists, elbows, and shoulders in the same manner, both hands together.
12. See this person turn their neck in all positions and directions.
13. See this person flex the jaw, wiggle the ears, and cut the eyes all around.

Visualizing in this way activates the centers in the brain which are responsible for joint movement. Your visualization of someone else activates your own center. It improves the action of the brain center itself and improves connection between the brain and the joints. The joints become more flexible. It is recommended to do mind exercises for the joints once a day for 10-30 minutes.

Important Note: Besides the mind exercises, it is necessary to also perform 15-20 minutes per day of real (physical) exercises for the joints, which are doable for you and do not cause you any pain. You may do simple yoga exercises as well.

Some Disorders and Illnesses Which Could Be Solved with Joint Cleansing

Joint pain, back pain, arthritis, rheumatoic arthritis, stiffness in joints, insomnia, etc.

Self-Testing
During Joint Cleansing

Does it Hurt?

If during joint cleansing procedure you feel pain in a certain area, it means that it is being intensively cleansed. Usually that pain does not last too long. If the pain or discomfort are not present at all, you are still having a successful cleansing, only not as intense. Special joint cleansing herbs and fresh juices you drink during that time, as well as warm, salt baths and FIR Sauna, dissolve uric acid and excrete it through different pathways: large intestine, skin and kidneys.

See what is being released through the kidneys:

Collect all your night and morning urine into a large (3 qt.) glass jar for a 2-4 weeks. Once the jar gets full, take another one, but make sure to label the jars with days (for instance, Days 1-2 or Days 2-4, etc). Store the jars in the dark cool place for 3 to 4 weeks. Within that time dissolved crystals of uric acid will crystalize again and drop to the bottom of the jar. It will look like small sand particles. You will also see a large quantity of mucus, which accumulates around the joints in the muscle tissue. In order to see sand and mucus in the glass jar, it is best to put it to the light or you can place a lamp behind the jar. You can also strain the urine through cheesecloth into another jar. After the liquid passes through the cloth, all the crystals and mucus will stay in the cloth. What you see is only a part of your joint toxicity. Large portion of toxicity will also be released through the skin and large intestine. It is recommended to follow joint cleansing procedure by kidney cleansing procedure, to completely remove toxins accumulated in the filters (kidneys).

What happens after?

After joint cleansing your joint and back problems will drastically improve or completely disappear and body's flexibility will increase. For those who suffer from arthritis or other joint problems, it is necessary to repeat the cleansing 3-5 times with 1-3 months intervals. Then, it is ideal to repeat the cleanse for maintenance once per year.

Test your joints.

You can test your joints way before you start getting any joint disorders or problems. If you do not use your joints' capabilities to the fullest, uric acid starts accumulating in the joints and toxic fluids retain in the muscle tissue around the joints. Blood circulation in the joints impairs. When joint movement lessens, also lessens flexibility of back and neck.

Can you do it?

Try these exercises:
1. Try to clasp your hands behind your back. Put one arm behind your back from the top (as if you are trying to scratch your upper back) and the other arm from the bottom as if you are trying to scratch your mid back. Then switch

the arms. How close did you get? Were both sides the same or different?

2. Touch the floor with your hands without bending knees,
3. Standing on your knees bend back and reach for your heels.

Do these simple exercises cause you any pain? Are you able to do them at all?

Do not let it happen!

In order not to allow salt accumulation in the joints and spine, you should do exercise for the joints on daily basis. Take hot baths with salt 1-2 times per week. Periodically do cleanses of joints and other organs.

SELF HELP: <u>*JOINT MAINTENANCE*</u>

Cover 2 table spoons of brown rice with cold, clean water. Put in a dark place over night or for 24 hours. In the morning, wash the rice, cover with clean water, cook and then eat. After that, do not eat or drink anything for 2-4 hours. Repeat again within 1-2 months.

"...Arthritis pain for over 20 years and finally relief! Doing all other cleanses to prepare for joint cleansing, made me feel better and better, but the Joint Cleanse itself made a huge difference. My knees are not swollen. My knuckles are shrinking before my eyes. I am able to exercise again and my flexibility is much better. I feel young and rejuvenated again and all I have to do to keep it up is to follow Dr. Koyfman's diet, exercise and other recommendations..."   *Lucy J.*

Step #6

Kidney Cleansing

"Helping your heart
and your sexuality."

Improve Health and Live Longer

The kidneys are important to your health because
this pair of organs filters harmful wastes from the fluids
circulating in your body, and sends these wastes to the
bladder for elimination.

If the kidneys are not working properly, wastes
remain in the body and poison it. The immune system has to
work that much harder to fight these unwanted chemicals.
Once these dangerous chemicals are flushed from your
body, they cannot continue to stress your immune system.

The kidneys also regulate the level of minerals in the
body and your acid-alkaline balance. When we do not drink
enough water or fresh, raw juices, our fluid levels fall too
low. Minerals build up in the kidneys and kidney stones can
form. The kidneys, overworked from mineral deposits,
become less efficient and effective. Dysfunction of the
kidneys is often the reason for pain in the lower part of the
back.

Experts have estimated that a minimum of 3,300,000 Americans do not realize that they have kidney disease. More than 20 million Americans suffer from kidney disease and urinary tract disease while some 80,000 will die of these two diseases in this country this year. It is estimated that 400,000 Americans have kidney stones. And kidney disease does not respect any age group.

Therefore, it is very wise to cleanse the kidneys from the wastes and minerals that have accumulated during a lifetime of eating processed food and food additives (unnatural chemicals) and inhaling various chemicals in our environment. Fortunately, this can be done in a safe and gentle manner using only natural techniques and foods.

Benefits of Kidney Cleansing

- Cleansing the blood, lymph system, ureters, and pancreatic gland plus both kidneys.
- Flushing away "sand," non-organic salt, mucous, kidney stones, and retained fluids.
- Increase the health and functioning of these organs and systems, plus the heart and other organs.
- Toxic weight, swelling in the legs, joint pain, and spine pain might disappear.
- Flexibility will be increased.
- Greater sexual satisfaction, since sexual energy comes from the kidneys.

For best results kidney cleansing should be done after Colon Cleansing and Complex Liver Cleansing. Depending on the kidney condition, this cleansing can be done over time from one week to one month.

Instructions
for
Kidney Cleansing

For those who are doing Kidney Cleansing as a preventative measure, in order to eliminate sand, small non-organic mineral salt crystals, and mucus, the program will require seven to ten days.

For those who have kidney stones, it may be necessary to repeat this program two or three times, depending on the size and number of these stones. In order to cleanse the kidneys from stones, non-organic mineral salt crystals and mucus, the following conditions must be met:

1. First decrease, and then maintain, a low level of pressure from fecal matter and gases in the abdominal area. High pressure in this area pushes down on the urethra, kidneys and other organs, inhibiting their function and cleansing. This decrease in pressure can be achieved by colon hydrotherapy, and by fasting or eating only small amounts of easily digestible food.

2. Drink a large amount of liquids, such as special juices and herbal extracts. These liquids are capable of dissolving stones and diluting mucous, washing them out of the kidneys.

3. In order to dislodge stones from where they are lodged, it is necessary to perform exercises such as walking, light jogging, or jumping on a miniature trampoline.

4. To improve the movement of stones through the urethra, the insides of its channels have to be lubricated. Foods which contain lubricant are flax seed and Ghee (clarified butter). Additionally, warm, natural oils rubbed on during a therapeutic massage, can serve as lubricants.

5. During Kidney Cleansing, the workload of the kidney is greatly increased. Whole body massages, reflexotherapy and kidneys massages help the kidneys handle their workload during that time. Also, the Cleansing Sauna, which helps eliminate toxins through the skin, takes a large amount of pressure off the kidneys.

6. It is very important that all channels of the urinary system can be easily widened in order to let big stones through. To achieve this, the body needs to be warmed both internally and externally. This is done by daily warm baths with salts and herbs, and also by drinking hot herbal extracts.

7. Certain Yoga exercises help to activate blood circulation through the kidneys, making them stronger and improving cleansing. These exercises include "The Locust," "The Bow," and "The

Cobra." If you are not familiar with these exercises, you may read about them in a book of yoga.

Sample Daily Schedule During Kidney Cleansing

1. After getting up, take a warm shower. Instead of using the towel, dry yourself by using your hands to rub the water off, for about 5 minutes.

2. Massage yourself with a dry brush for approximately 5 minutes.

3. Drink one cup of hot herbal tea, such as rose hips, parsley, or dandelion root, with half a teaspoon of Ghee.

4. Put your clothes on and do a few yoga exercises to activate kidneys.

5. If you have time take a 30 to 60 minute walk. Dress warmly if it's cold or windy.

6. If you have a trampoline jump for 5 to 10 minutes.

7. Before noon, you should consume 3 or 4 glasses of juice in the following proportions:
    Carrots -   10 oz.
    Cucumbers -   3 oz.
    Beats -   3 oz.

8. From 12 to 5 p.m., eat watermelon or drink watermelon juice as much as desired.

9.   For those who do not wish to lose weight, it is permitted to have a light dinner at 5 or 6 p.m. The amount of food should not exceed 6 to 8 oz. Alternatives for dinner:

      a.   Fresh salad of carrots, cucumber, lettuce, celery and lemon juice.

      b.   Vegetable soup.

      c.   Variety of steamed vegetables.

10.   One or one-and-one-half hours after dinner, drink hot herbal tea (rose hips, parsley, or dandelion root), with juice from ½ lemon. Stop drinking one hour before going to bed.

11.   Every day, for 15-30 minutes, take a warm bath with sea salt, between 5 p.m. and 9 p.m.

12.   To create internal lubrication:

      a.   Drink hot tea with ½ to 1 tsp. Ghee dissolved in it, 1 or 2 times a day.

      b.   Mix 1 glass of water with 1 tsp. flaxseed, heat to boiling, let stand for 10 minutes, and strain. Drink ½ glass twice a day, diluting with water.

Recommended Procedures During Kidney Cleansing

1.   Colon Cleansing
2.   FIR on the kidneys
3.   Kidney Massage with GX-99
4.   Far Infrared Sauna

5.   If possible, full body massage is also highly recommended.

* Special equipment called FIR is used to activate cellular blood circulation and to facilitate the elimination of stones and other toxins from the kidneys. It also helps to remove heavy metals from the body through the kidneys.

Some Disorders and Illnesses Which could Be Solved with Kidney Cleansing

Water retention, swollen joints, kidney stones, prostate problems, sexual problems, heart problems, lower back pain, heavy metal poisoning, ...

Testimonial: *Kidney stones, sex drive, energy*

"...passing that kidney stone was not exactly fun, but I am glad I did it without surgery or other strange medical procedures and medications. Dr. Koyfman's technique is very gentle and doable for anyone. Even before I got to the actual kidney cleansing, doing all the preparation cleanses made me feel much better. I did not have so much discomfort and pain in my kidneys. My sex life had improved drastically. I had more energy, etc. During my actual kidney cleansing, I started passing sand and small stones. Because of the good preparation the stones were mostly dissolved and broken down into small particles, which helped me pass them much easier. I am so glad I chose this method. I am a new man!"   Bob C.

Self-Testing
During Kidney Cleansing

The kidneys are designed to separate toxins from the body's fluids and eject them from the body. So kidneys are a part of the system's cleansing organs.

Food and Kidney Function.

Consuming excess amounts of salt, spice and sugars makes the body retain extra amounts of water to neutralize high concentration of these damaging elements. Excess fluid accumulates in the cells near joint tissue, muscles and organs, including kidneys themselves. By retaining extra water, cells stretch and increase in size losing their elasticity and cleansing abilities. Unfriendly bacteria and infection begin to accumulate and reproduce in the retained cellular fluid. Up to few pounds of toxic fluid can be accumulated just in kidneys. It causes kidneys to malfunction and not completely cleanse the body and themselves. By excess consumption of meat, dairy products, improper food combining and lack of movement– sand, stones, toxic mucus and undigested proteins and inorganic minerals ascend in the kidneys.

What can you see?

In order to see what is being released during your kidney cleansing, you can use the following technique. Collect all your night and morning urine into a large (3 qt.) glass jar for a week. Once the jar gets full, take another one, but make sure to label the jars with days (for instance, Days 1-2, Days 3-4, etc). Store the jars in the dark cool place for 3 to 4 weeks and then look it at it in the light. You can also strain it through the cheesecloth into a different dish. You will find sand, small stones and of course mucus on the surface of the cheesecloth. If desired, you may use a magnifying glass for more detailed observation.

Regular cleansing of kidneys (not less than 1 time per year), will improve function of the heart; help with hypertension; ease the workload for lungs; help or prevent reproductive organs dysfunctions; improve sex drive; extend your life.

SELF HELP Recipe: *KIDNEY MAINTENANCE*

Make juice: 12oz of carrot, 4 oz of beet, 4 oz of cucumber and 2 lemons. Mix the juice all together. Divide into 3 parts. Drink 3 times/day 20-30 minutes before meal for 7 days.

* For all kidney problems or disorders:

Avoid salty and spicy foods. Eat watermelon as often as possible. Drink diuretic teas, such as rose hips. Regularly do special kidney exercises from my book "Healing Through Cleansing 1".

Step #7

Lymph Cleansing

"Increasing the
strength of your
immune system."

What Is the Lymph System?

When you eat food, your body digests that food for
its nutrients, and then sends those nutrients to every living
cell in your body. As the cells consume these nutrients some
waste is created. The waste from each cell must be removed
or the body will "drown" in its own waste. The lymph
system, located throughout your body, provides the
"highway" by which this waste is transported from the cells
to the blood to the colon and kidneys. The lymph system
acts as a miniature sewer system.

Why Does the Lymph System Need Cleansing?

The lymph system is more than a transportation
system composed of lymphatic fluids. It also works as a
filter, removing bacteria, microorganisms, dead cells, and
other unwanted substances. Unfortunately, our bodies have

an abundance of these unwelcome substances which can block the lymph nodes, decreasing the body's ability to resist disease. Whenever the lymph system is overwhelmed by these toxic materials, or whenever the lymphatic filters become clogged (especially during illness) the system stores toxic mucous.

The lymph system is similar to the pipes that carry waste in a house. Over time, wastes build up on the insides of the pipe walls and start to clog the system. The same thing happens in the lymph system. Toxic mucous and other wastes build up in the lymph system and hinder its function.

Because the lymph system is a part of the immune system, it is vital that its function not be hindered by useless wastes that can be naturally flushed out. There is a domino effect of good health for the entire body if this system is kept clean and healthy. Otherwise chronic illness of various types can result.

How Can the Lymph System Be Cleansed?

Fortunately, the lymph system can be stimulated to release its wastes in a natural, gentle way, and at the same time to replace its own lymphatic fluids.

The best results are achieved after a full Complex Liver Cleansing. For Lymph Cleansing, the Center uses mineral salt and/or juice therapy, lymphatic massage, and Colon Cleansing. A highly concentrated mineral salt solution consumed in the morning creates a reverse osmosis condition in the body, attracting the old lymph fluids to the mineral salt solution. The old lymph fluids pass through the intestinal walls and are eliminated with the feces and urine. Fresh juices absorb well at this time, and their biologically active water replaces the old and dirty lymph fluids.

What Benefits Will I Receive from a Lymph Cleansing?

- Rejuvenates the white blood cells.
- Stimulates such glands the liver, pancreas, etc.
- Improves digestion.
- Cleanses the kidneys, ureters and joints.
- Increases immunity.
- Helps the body fight diseases.
- Cleanses the blood and blood vessels.

Who Needs a Lymph Cleanse?

Everyone needs to have his or her lymph system cleansed from all the wastes that have built up over a lifetime. Cleansing this important system of the body helps to cleanse every organ and system you have. The Lymph Cleansing offered by the Center has far reaching health effects because the lymph system reaches into every part of the body.

When Should I Have My Lymph System Cleansed?

For the best results, you should first do: Colon Cleansing, Whole Digestive System, Complete Small Intestine, Complex Liver Cleansing and Kidney Cleansing.

Instructions
for
Lymph Cleansing

"Laying the
foundation . . . day of
dedication."

In order to maximize the results of Lymph
Cleansing, it is necessary first to cleanse the large intestine
(colon), the whole digestive system, and the liver.

However, if personal circumstances do not permit
Colon Cleansing and Complex Liver Cleansing to be
completed first, then Lymph Cleansing can still be
beneficial. In this case it would be best to do the Lymph
Cleansing three days in a row, or if necessary, every other
day for three days.

If one is able to complete Colon Cleansing, Whole
Digestive System Cleansing, and Complex Liver Cleansing
before cleansing the lymph, then the time between Lymph
Cleansings can be a week or two.

For Lymph Cleansing, **preparation is a must. If it
has been more than ten days since you did any kind of
cleansing, Lymph Cleansing is not permitted.**

How Many Procedures Are Required for Lymph Cleansing?

The amount of lymphatic and other fluids in the body is approximately twelve liters. During one day of lymphatic cleansing, about four liters of lymphatic fluid are exchanged. (*Lymph fluids have a light yellow and white color. Juices change the color.*) Therefore, full Lymph Cleansing, or full fluid exchange, requires three procedures. Usually, for maintaining health and preventing disease, Lymph Cleansing should be done once every one to three years, depending on the person's health condition and other cleansing programs. If necessary, Lymph Cleansing can be repeated after one to three months.

Two / Three Days Before the Lymph Cleansing

1. Eat only a vegetarian diet for two to three days prior to Lymph Cleansing with the main accent on fresh fruits and vegetables, freshly made organic fruit and vegetable juices, clean distilled water in large enough amount, whole grains, soups, etc.
2. Take a warm bath once a day for two or three days prior to Lymph Cleansing. Use herbs (sage, camomile) and sea salt in the water, and keep the atmosphere relaxing.
3. Obtain whatever kitchen items you may need such as: Citrus juicer - quality is important
    Cutting boards - large, impermeable
    Strainers - the finer the mesh the better
    Large glass or ceramic pitcher is preferred but can be substituted with good quality plastic.

One Day Before the Lymph Cleansing

The citrus fruits you will need are:
- **10-12 organic oranges**
- **8-10   organic grapefruits**
- **5-8   organic lemons**
- **2 liters of clean, distilled water**

Please note that **these are approximate amounts.** You may need more depending on the "juiciness" of the citrus fruits available in your local area. You may also need more depending on your personal body size. Larger persons have more lymphatic fluid and therefore need to replace a larger volume. Also, try to purchase citrus fruits that are medium-sized and properly ripe. (This is a good time to support your local health food grocery store.)

If you are allergic to any of the above citrus fruits, you will have to substitute carrots and celery. In this case you will need to buy:
- **30-40 organic carrots**
- **10-20 organic celery sticks**
- **2 liters of clean, distilled water**

Again, please note that **these are approximate amounts.**

Keep these foods (either citrus fruits or vegetables) at room temperature until you wash and peel them a day before the Lymph Cleansing. Then **refrigerate** them.

On the Day of the Lymph Cleansing

Clean and organize your kitchen so that nothing will interfere with the healthiness and ease of your preparations.

Set out all the kitchen utensils you will need:

- Citrus juicer
- Cutting boards
- Strainers
- Pitcher
- Sharp kitchen knives
- Clean glasses

You will make freshly squeezed citrus juice. The proportion of orange to grapefruit to lemon is 4.5:4.5:1. It is better to make this juice throughout the day as opposed to all at once. This will help retain the vitality of the juices. Also, all of these juices must be strained through a very fine strainer or few layers of cheesecloth to remove seeds and pulp. All measurements of juice volume must be done after straining.

Recipe for Biologically Active Drink for the Renewal of Lymphatic Fluids

10-12 oranges	900 ml. juice	4 cups
6-8-10 grapefruits	900 ml. juice	4 cups
4-5-8 lemons	200 ml. juice	1 cup
Total:	2000 ml. juice	9 cups

Once this juice has been made, store it in a glass or ceramic pitcher in your refrigerator. **It is important to keep all fresh juices cool and away from light to preserve their vitamins and minerals.** Cover the pitcher tightly with plastic wrap to limit further air circulation inside the pitcher of juice.

Also, do not mix the juices with water until immediately before drinking. Otherwise chemical reactions will occur that will hinder the effectiveness of the juices.

Optional Recipe for Lymphatic Renewal Drink

30-40 carrots	1500 ml. juice	6.5 cups
10-20 celery sticks	500 ml. juice	2.5 cups
Total:	2000 ml. juice	9 cups

The same recommendations apply to these vegetable juices: both of these **juices must be strained** to remove pulp, the mixture must be stored in a glass or ceramic pitcher in the refrigerator until use, and do not mix the juices with water until immediately before drinking. *All measurements of juice volume must be done after straining.*

1.   **Prepare the juices from the recipe above.** (*Make the juices, strain them, and put them immediately in the refrigerator.*)

2.   When you finish making the juices, **drink the solution provided by the Center.** The solution should be kept in the refrigerator as well. Then, before you start, you will **warm the solution to body temperature** as described for juices below. If you do not warm the solution and your juices to body temperature, you may get sick during the Lymph Cleanse. This solution "jump starts" the cleansing process. If the taste of the solution is unpleasant, take two or three sips of clean water, or suck (*but not swallow*) a piece

of orange or grapefruit.

The high concentration of natural salt in the solution creates an osmotic effect in the body (the passage of a "solvent" from a less concentrated to a more concentrated solution through a semipermeable membrane). The highly concentrated salt solution draws to itself the less concentrated fluid—the lymph—through the walls of the digestive system. This solution may also have a laxative effect, so you will want to stay within easy access of a toilet for the morning, and perhaps the afternoon. It will usually take 30 to 45 minutes, sometimes up to two hours, to create the urge to go to the bathroom.

3. Right after drinking the solution, **take a warm bath or shower** for 15 to 20 minutes. The moist heat of the warm bath begins and enhances the process of pulling old lymphatic fluids and associated toxins into the digestive system, through which they are sent to the colon and kidneys.

4. After the warm bath, **begin to drink the juice/water** mixture prepared earlier. **The time frame between the solution you drank and your first juice/water, should not exceed 30 minutes.** Mix the juices and the distilled water "fifty-fifty" in the following manner:

    a. Shake the juice container to stir its contents.
    b. Pour 4 oz. (100 g.) of juice into a glass.
    c. Put the container of juice back in the refrigerator immediately.
    d. Pour 4 oz. (100 g.) of distilled water into the glass with the juice.
    e. **Warm the juice/water mixture gently to body**

temperature in a pan of hot water (see below).

f.   Drink it with moderate speed.

Please note: If you experience itching, this means that you are allergic to this juice. You must immediately stop drinking it and switch to carrot and celery juice.

5.   You should repeat this process every 20-30 minutes until you finish all the juice. If you have not finished all of the juice/water mixture by the time of your appointment at the Center, please bring it with you. You will finish drinking it when you come to the Center.

    Important Consideration: Please remember this about the biologically active, diluted juice you are drinking: It is absorbed by the body and exchanged for the old toxic lymph. **These juices are the raw material from which your new lymphatic fluids are made**. Because of this, you want the highest quality fruit (or vegetable) juices possible. **Canned juices or other purchased/prepared juices are biologically dead and filled with artificial ingredients.** Who would want to use such unnatural, pre-poisoned material to create new lymph fluids? Stick with making your own juices from organically grown produce, and making them just before using them. Remember that light and heat damage the vitality of the juices, so put them in the refrigerator to keep them cool and away from light. Also cover the pitcher tightly with plastic wrap to limit further air circulation inside the pitcher of juice.

    How to warm the juice/water mixture slowly:
Warm water in a pan until it is very warm but not hot. Place the glass containing the juice/water mixture into the warm water. Mix the juice solution periodically with a spoon.

Take a drop from the solution periodically, and put on the back of the hand, to check its temperature. **Do not let the juice/water mixture get hot.**

In the first three or four hours, the cleansing will come through the large intestine (colon). Then the process will change, and the cleansing will continue through the kidney in the form of urine.

Each day the Lymph Cleansing consists of home procedures and office procedures. Whether you are at home or the office first during the day is equally effective and will be discussed when you schedule your Lymph Cleansing.

Services Provided at the Center

1.   *Lymphatic Massage (Drainage)* This service is done by using two pieces of state-of-the-art equipment:

a.   **GX-99.** This machine uses mechanical vibrations at a frequency of between 30 and 50 millihertz to stimulate the lymph system to release old lymph fluids. The GX-99 helps to clean the lymphatic ducts and activate the flowing of lymphatic fluids in the muscles and internal organs. The use of this machine has at least two side benefits:
    • Slimming the body.
    • Lessening the cellulite.
You don't have to be enrolled in any program to enjoy the benefits of the GX-99.

b. **The Lymphstar Pro.** This machine uses light energy on the tender parts of the body where major lymph nodes are located. The Lymph Pro machine helps to clean the lymph nodes of the neck, armpits, groin, and breast areas. The use of this machine also has additional benefits:

- Risk reduction for breast cancer.
- Risk reduction for lymph cancer.
- Risk reduction for blood cancer.

The Lymphstar Pro machine: uses neon light which passes through the skin and causes the molecules of blood and lymph to separate in the lymph system. This eases the transition of the old, toxic lymphatic fluids, relieves soreness in the lymph nodes and increases oxygen flow to prevent tissues from becoming hard.

2. *Cleansing of the Large Intestine.* The Center uses Colon Cleansing (colon hydrotherapy) to gently flush out the rest of the toxic lymphatic fluids in order to prevent their reabsorption in the colon.

3. *Infrared Sauna.* The Cleansing Infrared Sauna activates and supports the function of the eliminating organs, such as the liver and kidneys, drawing toxins from the lymph system and the rest of the body, and removing them through the skin by perspiration.

During this day, you probably will not have any desire to eat. But if you feel hungry at the end of the day, it is permissible to eat some oranges or grapefruit or *carrots and celery* (depending on which juice you drank earlier). Also, you may drink clean water, or eat a small amount of vegetarian food like fresh salad.

Your Diet After the Lymph Cleansing

For the next three days after your Lymph Cleansing, your food must be 80-100% raw. This includes fresh fruits, vegetables, and their juices. Ten to twenty percent of your food could be steamed vegetable, vegetable soups, or cooked whole grains.

Therapeutic Effect of Lymph Cleansing and Lymphatic Drainage

Your Lymph Cleansing will provide you with the following benefits:
- Cleansed lymphatic system.
- Brand-new lymphatic fluids
- Cleansed blood vessels and blood.
- Cleansed kidneys.
- Cleansed skin.
- Increased immunity and resistance to many diseases.
- Improved blood quality.
- Activation of the hormonal glands.
- Improved digestion.

For those who may need to repeat Lymph Cleansing, it is advised to alternate the choice of juices. If you choose citrus the first time, then switch to carrot/celery for the next time, and vice versa.

Some Disorders and Illnesses Which Could be Solved with Lymph Cleansing

Swollen lymph nodes, skin problems, high cholesterol, constipation, headaches, colds, sinus problems, weak immune system, chronic fatigue, ...

SELF HELP: *SUPER LYMPH CLEANSER*

Lymph Cleansing Beverage.
Mix together:
4oz of beet juice
4oz of carrot juice
4oz of honey
4 oz of vodka
To consume:
mix 2 table spoons of the solution in 4 oz of water and take 3 times/ day before meals, until the whole jar is gone.

Also see book Healing Through Cleansing 3 for daily lymph cleansing techniques. Periodically, repeat herbal parasite cleansing to kill infection.

Self-Testing
During the Lymph Cleansing

The Blood

The main function of the blood is to deliver nutrients to the cells of the body. When nutrients reach the cells, they undergo a "cellular digestion", in the result of which some toxic elements are formed.

The Lymph

The main function of the lymphatic system is to evacuate accumulated toxins from the cells, neutralize them in the lymph nodes and eliminate them from the body through cleansing channels: kidneys, skin, lungs and large intestine. Because lymphatic system neutralizes and eliminates toxicity on the cellular level, it serves a protective function and is a big part of the Immune System.

Lymphatic System consists of lymphatic fluid, lymph nodes, tonsils and spleen. Most people do not realize the importance of tonsils. There are three pairs of tonsils. One pair is on the root of the tongue, second is on the both sides of the throat and third (adenoids) are located at the point where throat and sinus passages connect.

Tonsils are our body's first line of defense from exterior toxicity and are subject to chronic infections. When they get filled with bacteria and infection, they swell up and hurt. Many people have them removed leaving their bodies without any protection from exterior. Lymph cleansing procedure would cleanse the tonsils naturally, remove the

129

infection and repair their functioning of these important glands.

Spleen, in medical field is considered as something unnecessary for adult body. It is not really the case. Spleen serves an important role and is a big part of the immune system. It is an "emergency blood bank" for the body, which holds more than a pint (500 ml) of blood and releases it into the system when needed. The spongy like tissue of the spleen is one of the major filters for the lymphatic fluid. As any filter, it gets filled with toxicity and can become infected itself. In that case, it can either be surgically removed or cleansed naturally by doing a lymph cleansing procedure. A research exists that individuals who have their spleen removed, most likely, will not live past 50 years of age.

The Cleansing

In our Center, cleansing and elimination of old, toxic lymphatic fluid goes through three main channels– large intestine, kidneys and skin. These channels release all types of accumulated toxins:
- External toxins which enter from air, water and food..
- Internal toxins resulting from bad digestion, stress and aging.
- Toxic chemicals from food, beverages and medicines.
- Heavy metals, toxic mucus, inorganic salts and much more

To see these wastes in the process of the lymph cleansing is not that easy, because lymphatic toxicity and intestinal waste release together. To determine the actual lymphatic waste, it is necessary to pay close attention to what is being released in the restroom and what it smells like. This careful observation will give you an idea of how clean or toxic your lymphatic fluid really is. If you have done self-testing in the previous procedures and learned to distinguish colon, small intestine and liver wastes, by the time you do your lymph cleansing, you should be an expert and should be able to tell what is what.

By cleansing the lymph through the large intestine, you also cleanse the whole digestive system. That is why toxicity of digestive system and lymphatic toxicity will be mixed together. Lymphatic toxicity contains an enormous amount of mucus, which is full of heavy metals, chemical elements, bacteria, infections, etc.

To observe toxicity in the urine, you may collect all the urine you release during the three day process of the lymph cleansing. Let it sit about a week or longer and then observe it. You may see more toxic mucus in it than anything else.

Please understand, that no matter what you see coming out of you, lymphatic cleansing will make your immune system and health much stronger. Keep the achieved success by following a healthy life style. Remember, it is easier to damage your health, than to repair it.

Step #8

Cell Cleansing (Fasting)

"The Ph.D. of natural healing, helping you reach optimal health and look younger."

How Do Cells Accumulate Waste?

The organs of the human body are made up of tissues, which in turn are made up of billions of individual cells. When we eat food, the stomach, small intestine, and large intestine digest the food in order to separate nutrients (vitamins, minerals, proteins, etc) from unusable materials (waste). The nutrients are then sent to every part of the body to feed these cells.

As the nutrients are "burned" at the cellular level, waste is created within the cells that (too often) is not completely removed. As time passes and cells are replaced, the waste products are left behind within the tissues of that organ. These toxic wastes poison the cells, weakening them and making them susceptible to illness and disease.

The question now is how to gently coax the body, on a cellular level, to release these wastes and thereby strengthen the immune system. The answer lies in proper fasting, preferably under the supervision of a trained professional who can maximize the health benefits of the fast through centuries-proven techniques.

Solving the Problem

When we stop eating, the body seeks to obtain energy anywhere it can. Since no new sources of energy or food are coming in from the outside, it will search around for what it can consume that is already present on the inside of the body.

The human body is incredibly wise when it comes to healing itself, so it naturally avoids consuming any part of itself that is necessary or useful to its own health. Therefore, it begins by eating or consuming dead cells, dying cells, sick cells, and fat cells first.

With its attention now focused on identifying which cells constitute fuel, it begins to recognize more clearly those cells that it cannot consume and that the body cannot use. "House Cleaning" begins in a vigorous and determined way.

The body begins to dump any unhealthy materials such as toxic mucous, tumor and cancer cells, different kinds of salts, cholesterol, the chemical dregs of any kind of drugs, nicotine, and other stagnated matter which is stored in the tissues and organs. The body also disposes of the unseen toxic weight stored inside.

All cleansings, except fasting, cleanse only the internal surface of the organ and its inner passageways where materials have accumulated in masses of various sizes. While these other (valuable) cleansings remove large percentages of accumulated waste, they are unable to reach into the cellular level. Or shall we say, the regular cleansing "cleans the house," but cellular cleansing "sweeps the corners."

The philosophy (and reality) of this is that all toxins in the body decrease your health. The regular cleansings (described in preceding chapters) get the vast majority of toxins, and therefore will strengthen your immune system, lengthen your life, and improve the quality of life. But with cellular cleansing, the remainder of your body's toxins can be removed, thereby taking your immune system to the zenith of its strength, providing the longest life your body can achieve, and maximizing your quality of life.

Fasting

Fasting, by itself, is not enough to truly cleanse the billions of cells of the body. Although critically important to this procedure, it still needs a little help.

The Center maximizes the natural flushing action of the body during fasting with such techniques as a full body "healing massage," a cleansing sauna, and freshly made natural juices used in correct sequence and amount. During this time, the body is flushed with lots of clean water, while also given strategic, limited nourishment in the form of biologically active juices and organic herbal teas.

When these elements are synchronized under the trained eye of professionals with decades of experience, and tailored for your particular circumstance, the body fully activates the flushing out of toxins down to the cellular level, and with the least discomfort.

Once this process has begun during the fast, the body begins to "eat" its own diseases, harmful bacteria, unhealthy chemicals brought into the body, and toxins created in the body. Parasites that may be present weaken and sometimes die, and are then excreted. Fasting helps the body to dispose of toxic matter by supporting and cleansing all eliminating organs. The Center, in turn, supports the eliminating organs such as the skin (through Cleansing Sauna), the colon (through Colon Cleansing), and the other internal organs (through Cleansing Massage).

Does This Process Slow Down Aging?

On the cellular level, youth and aging are determined by the relative amount of old and young cells. In youth, the number of young, healthy, and strong cells predominates over the number of old, weak, and sick cells. With time, the cells become polluted and old, and the renewing ability of the body decreases.

During fasting, by switching from outer to inner nourishment, the body "eats" old and sick cells, and the body's ability to exchange old cells for new cells increases and speeds up. Metabolism improves.

During the breaking of the fast (the renewal period), the body replaces the "eaten" cells for new, healthy, young cells. At the Center, the renewal period is accompanied by healthy, specialized eating and special exercises. (Do not underestimate the importance how to break the fast. If done incorrectly, many, if not most, of the benefits of fasting can be destroyed.)

The person who does seasonal fasting regularly, without waiting for disease to come, looks so much younger than his or her age. This person is full of energy and has high resistance to disease.

What Kind of Fasting Is Used in Our Center?

We use the **Nourishing and Rejuvenative Fasting,** which is the easiest and least stressful kind of fasting.

During this kind of fasting, you will receive a detailed program, which allows you to drink clean water, herbal teas, fresh fruit juices, vegetable juices, and vegetable broth. If done correctly, one may also chew some vegetables without swallowing anything except the juice. (Inquire about Koyfman Fasting©.)

Will I Have Enough Energy to Continue Working During the Fast?

The Nourishing and Rejuvenative Fast puts the body on a high energy level. During the fasting, energy channels open up and become unclogged. Because of this, fasting promotes the body's reception of cosmic, earth, air, and sun energy. Energy is released and received from the "chewing" of the water, and the fruit and vegetable juices.

Therefore, the energy level of a fasting person is not lower than the energy level of the person who eats. Sometimes it is even higher.

Therapeutic Effects of Fasting

* Helps to lose visible weight.
* Cleanses the body on the cellular level.
* Helps the body to heal itself.
* Rejuvenates the body.

- Supports, strengthens, improves the immune system.
- Increases belief in one's own strength.
- Cleanses on the emotional and psychological levels.
- Improves digestion.
- Improves **metabolism**.
- Improves vision and hearing.
- Improves the skin condition.
- Gives the colon rest during the fast.
- Activates the work of the colon after the fast.
- Promotes active and healthy longevity.

Testimonials:

"...I thought it would be so difficult to fast. I thought I'd be hungry and week all the time, but I was amazed that I felt great all the time. First couple of days were harder, but then, it got easier every day..." R.T.

"...my thinking was never so clear. I was 10 days into the fast and I felt like I awakened. Everything looked, felt, smelled different. The life itself was more beautiful than ever. Answers to all my problems and concerns just kept coming in. It felt like I was connected to the Higher Forces..." L.M

"...I could not make myself stop the fast. I felt so light and clearheaded, I did not want to lose that feeling. Dr. Koyfman put me on a 21-day-fast, but I kept going for 140 days. I can't even describe how great I felt during the fast and what kind of difference it made for my body. I look at least 20 years younger..." B.M.

Instructions
for
Cell Cleansing (Fasting)

"A program of healing
and rejuvenating
fasting."

Preparation for the Fast

**To make fasting successful and yield the best
results, it is necessary to do all the steps properly.**
Three days prior to beginning the fast, stay on a strict
cleansing vegetarian diet: fruits, soaked dried fruits, fresh
fruit and vegetable juices, fresh salads, soups, grains, small
amounts of nuts and seeds soaked in water for 4-8 hours.

Entering the Fast

Often those who don't properly understand the
processes that happen in the body during fasting begin
fasting without any special care or plan, and without the
needed background knowledge. This is not wise.
During fasting, the system does not stop feeding; it
simply reorients its hunger during the fast to internal
feeding. If the fasting begins without complete cleansing of
the digestive system, then the body will spend a long time

feeding itself on leftover toxins and thereby poisoning itself. Such fasting is difficult for the person fasting. You may feel weakness, dizziness, nausea, or heart palpitations.

When fasting begins with a full cleansing of the various organs in the body, as described in the preceding chapters, then the body will not (cannot) waste its time and energy consuming toxins. It goes directly to feeding on old/dead/dying/sick cells. These cells go through the digestive process and are "digested" in the sense that what is useful is separated from what is not useful. (The healthy cells are left alone; the digestive process does not touch them.)

As these cells are burned in the fire of internal digestion, what nutrients are available feed the body, and the remainder (toxic mucus, excessive fat, tumors, cancer cells, etc) are sent out of the body via the excretory organs.

During such fasting some people can lose as much as 10 to 70 pounds of toxic weight, depending on personal circumstances. With this load of poisonous weight ("dead weight," pun intended) gone from the body, the healing and rejuvenation processes and shift into fifth gear.

The Role of the Liver in Fasting

The liver, ever the superstar of healing, plays a very important role during the fast. As useless cells are digested, it is the liver that neutralizes the toxins released by the digestion. If, before the fast, the liver is fully cleansed and in tip-top shape, it can better handle the work and make the fast easier to go through. **A day of Complex Liver Cleansing could be an entrance to the fast.**

So, if we combine Complex Liver Cleansing with the cleansing of the whole digestive system (Stomach, Colon and Small Intestine cleansings), fasting will be more effective, and you can go through the fast with ease and comfort. If one can not do all of these cleansings prior to fasting then, at a bare minimum, one should precede fasting with Colon Cleansing.

Important Procedures During the Fast

During the fast, and through the first week after you break the fast, you should consider doing any of the following combinations of procedures. **The more procedures you do the more toxins you expel and the better you feel.**

The most recommended procedures during the fast are Whole Digestive System Cleansing with FIR Sauna.
Your other options are:
- Colon Cleansing.
- Colon Cleansing with Internal Organ Massage.
- Colon Cleansing with sauna.
- Full body cleansing massage with a Colon Cleansing and sauna.

Doing the Fast Itself

This is a sample of a fasting schedule during the day. Depending on your personal and work schedule, plus any personal health problems, you can change it. Just keep in mind the main principles. (See section below entitled, "Important Principles of Fasting.")

7:00 a.m.   a.   In the morning after waking up, drink 1 to 2 glasses of warm, distilled water plus 1 tsp. strained lemon juice.

b.	Warm or contrast shower without soap.
c.	Dry skin brush massage, 3 to 5 minutes.
d.	Light morning exercise, 10 to 15 minutes.
e.	Outside walking, 20 minutes to 1 hour, with cleansing breathing technique (described in the book, *Healing through Cleansing,* in the chapter on the lungs).

9:00 a.m.   Big cup of warm herbal mint tea.

11:00 a.m.   Fruit juice: ½ cup juice (citrus, such as grapefruit, lemon, or orange, or apple) in ½ cup distilled water. **All juices on a fast must be strained**. This will prevent the stomach from having to work during the fast by digesting small food particles. It will also help to rest the colon. The juice will be absorbed directly by the small intestines.

1:00 p.m.   Vegetable juice (strained): 1 to 2 glasses.
- 60% choice of 2-3 kinds of green juices: celery, romaine lettuce, spinach, kale, cucumber, mustard and other greens.
- 40% juice from carrots, apples or pineapples.

3:00 p.m.   Warm herbal tea from rose hips or fasting tea.

| 5:00 p.m. | a. | Apple/beet juice: 4 apples plus 1/4 beet. |
| | b. | 1 to 2 glasses clean, distilled water. |

7:00 p.m. 1 to 2 cups warm, strained Potassium Vegetable Broth. (No substitute broth is allowed. See below for recipe.)

9:00 p.m. Warm herbal tea with camomile. May add ⅓ to ½ tsp. honey dissolved in tea. If you have yeast in your body, use stevia.

Walking before going to bed, 30 minutes. This is NOT power walking, but strolling *for relaxation,* so do not walk too fast.

Warm shower without soap. This is to increase circulation and not for exterior cleanliness. Shower or bathe for exterior cleanliness at a different time.

10:00-11:00 p.m. Go to bed no later than this time.

Recipe for Potassium Vegetable Broth:

Base: 1. Two big organic potatoes cut into cubes (1 cm.).
2. One glass shredded carrot.
3. One glass shredded beet.
4. One glass shredded celery (sticks or root).

Can be added: 1. One-half glass of cut onion.
2. Roots of parsley.
3. Beet tops.

Cover this with good clean water or previously distilled water, 1 or 2 cm. above the vegetables.

- Bring to a boil, then continue to simmer on low heat for 30 minutes.
- Turn off heat.
- Add upper green parts of beet, dill and parsley. Let stand for 30 minutes.
- Strain.
- While it is still warm, drink 1 or 2 eight-ounce cups.
- Put the rest in the refrigerator.

Important Note:

All teas, juices, broths must be strained and drunk warm or cool (never cold). Do not eat the solids.

It is very important to strain all juices and vegetable broth through a few (3 to 5) layers of cheesecloth, in order not to allow any pulp to get into the drink. If you drink anything that contains pulp, it is not fasting, it is a liquid diet. Your stomach will not stop working and the body will not get into the cellular cleansing mode.

If the juice you made is too sweet, dilute it with water in the proportion 3/4 of juice and 1/4 of water, or even 50/50 (half juice, half water). It is necessary to do to lower the concentration of sugar in the juice and prevent gas and feeding of yeast. If after adding the water, the juice became too sour, you may add a few drops of Stevia (a natural sweetener which does not feed yeast).

Attention clients with <u>YEAST</u> problem.

*You have to drink more of **green juices**: spinach, lettuce, cucumbers, celery, etc. It is also recommended to add 1-2 cloves of garlic per 1 glass of juice. **Garlic is wonderful remedy for yeast.** Throughout the day drink hot water with lemon, which will disinfect the digestive system, neutralize toxicity and kill yeast as well. It is also great to drink*
Onion Broth *throughout the day. Cut in cubes 1lb of onions. Cover with 2qrts. of water. Bring to a boil. Simmer for 10 minutes. Let stand for another 10 minutes. Strain well and drink warm. If you are at work, you may put it in the thermos to keep warm, otherwise refrigerate and then warmup.*

One woman in our Center was in her second three-week fast without receiving the expected benefits in energy and weight loss. We could not understand this until she mentioned that she used cubes of organic chicken broth instead of the recipe provided in this book.

Here are the reasons this is not allowed:

During this healing and rejuvenating fast, one must avoid fats, amino acids, and salt, which are items very present in pre-processed chicken broth, even if organic. Chicken soup may be a homemade remedy that works in certain instances, but this healing and rejuvenating fast follows a different principle of healing.

Further, ridding your body of disease and reversing the aging process are no small accomplishments. The fast that will be effective requires much work and a commitment

144

to be involved in your own healing. **Buying ready-made, pre-processed solutions will never suffice, even if they are organic and vegetable.**

Important Principles of Fasting

1. Wear clean clothes because they will help to accumulate more toxins from the skin. So change your clothes every single day. The underwear is the most important article of clothing here.
2. Use underwear made of natural fibers, not synthetic materials. Synthetic clothes accumulate negative electricity which can destroy body energies.
3. Wear extra clothing to stay warm since you might feel cold during a fast. If you have more clothes and don't feel cold, you save more energy for healing rather than wasting it for heating.
4. Before drinking anything, rinse your mouth with water, or water plus baking soda, or water and lemon juice.
5. During the day, try to find the time for walking 1 to 2 hours. During fasting, our bodies need more oxygen to neutralize the toxins.
6. Do a dry brush massage every morning and possibly every evening for 5-10 minutes.
7. Get some light exercise.
8. Try to stay calm, concentrate on yourself, not reacting to anything around you.
9. Try to find time for resting (not sleeping) with warm water bottle or heating pad on the right side for 30 to 60 minutes to heat your liver. (It will help your liver to detoxify itself and your whole body).
10. At any time, when you feel thirst, hunger or discomfort, drink distilled water.

11. Take a warm bath at least every other day, better every day. During fasting, the body cools down easily and cannot maintain the needed warm temperature (especially during cold weather). A warm bath helps to warm it up, stimulate circulation for toxin removal and to soak the toxins out. If you are doing a warm bath, you may skip #9 above.

12. Call the Center any time you feel you need support or help.

13. Don't break the fast without consulting with the Center. Breaking the fast when you are not feeling well involves a special program.

Tips to Remember

- Fasting cleanses and rejuvenates the whole body down to the cellular level.

- During fasting some people feel a slight discomfort, plus "flashbacks" to the feelings of old diseases and disorders, weakness, etc., as their stored remnants work themselves out. But all of this is for a short period of time, tolerable, and so much easier than the diseases themselves. These are called "healing events."

- If you feel bad, drink a cup of water with a pinch of sea salt to neutralize toxins (people who don't have yeast can add 1/3 teaspoon of honey).

- The benefits fasting brings are so amazing that it is worth the challenge.

- Look at this struggle as your fight with the sickness living inside you. In this fight you must win.

Caution: After you complete your fast, it is very important to break the fast correctly. Incorrect exiting from the fast may destroy all the benefits from your efforts as well as your health.
To find out how to break a fast, read the next chapter entitled, "Detailed Instructions for Exiting the Fast."

SELF HELP: _**SUPER BLOOD CLEANSER**_

Blood vessel cleansing recipe.
Wash thoroughly and grind together in the blender or in the meat grinder:
12 oz of dried apricots
12 oz of black raisins
12 oz walnuts
then add 12 oz honey
Mix well together and store in the refrigerator. Take for 6 months in the morning on empty stomach.
Men- 1 tablespoon.
Women- 1 medium spoon (smaller than a tablespoon, larger than a teaspoon).

Self-Testing
During Cell Cleansing (Fasting)

What can you see during the cellular cleansing?

Methods of dissolving cellular toxicity and its elimination from the body during fasting are: drinking an adequate amount of fresh juices, good water and herbal teas; FIR sauna; cleansing of the whole digestive system; long walks, etc.

You will mainly see the elimination of that toxicity in the restroom during your Whole Digestive System cleansing procedure. Cellular toxicity differs from others by a darker color, stronger smell and more mucus, which overfills the body of any modern person. This release does not happen daily. The body first needs to gather-up enough of that toxicity and only then it can release it. With each of these strong eliminations you cleanse a new portion of cells, remove not only toxicity, but also illnesses that come with it.

How do you feel during Fasting?

If you went through the complete cleansing of the digestive system and liver cleansing, and entered the fast correctly, you should mainly feel good during the fast, or sometimes even better than when you eat. You should be absolutely capable of working and doing all your daily functions just like before the fast.

However, there will be some hours (or sometimes a full day) when your energy level would drop. You would want to lay down and not doing anything at all. You might also notice an increase in old pains and discomforts, which were long forgotten or you never knew of. Some individuals get scared at the moments like these and feel an urge to break the fast.

What happens in your body during those tough moments?

Why do you feel fatigue and other problems? Why does the willpower drop and you get scared? Why do you want to start eating?

This period is very important during the fast. During this time you may receive answers to these and other questions. You just have to ask yourselves before making any drastic decisions. You may wonder what is the point to ask yourself questions you do not have the answers. When you ask yourself a question and patiently wait for an answer-turn on your intuition, unconsciousness and logic, and answers slowly start to come. Repeat the question over and over again and just wait. You will get the answer.

I can provide you with some main answers and reasons why you might feel these discomforts while fasting. The more detailed answers can only be known by you.

Feeling fatigue– it means that your body found a serious problem and is putting all its strength into liquidating it. Since most energy at that time is being used internally, you do not have much of it to use externally. Of course you can make yourself do something, but that would not be wise because you will take part of that energy, which is vital to fight the problem. So at times like that, it is best not to do anything and allow yourself to lay down and relax for at least a short period of time.

Fear, loss of willpower and need for food– is a result of unhealthy bacteria, viruses, infection and other parasites, which also feel hunger during your fast because of lack of fresh foods and flushed out toxic wastes. Their lives are under threat and their powers drop as well. Due to these circumstances, their body releases elements/signals, which cause discomforts in your body (such as a need to eat, lack of wheel power and fear).

If you give in to the panic and begin to eat, you will save the lives of creatures living inside of you and stop the process of healing and rejuvenation of your body. So decision is yours- to save yourselves or the parasites.

Why does the pain increase?

In order to liquidate pain and problem, it is necessary for your body to get to the root of the illness or disorder and "rip it out" from the system with its roots. The process of "ripping off the roots" is the cause of the pain. Luckily that process is not long and pain goes away quickly within few hours, or in extreme cases 1-2 days. However, from that point on, that pain should not bother you again.

Why does new pain emerge? Pain you might never experienced before.

Emersion of new pain means that the body found and started healing of the problems, which began to develop in your body, but never got to the "surface" and you never knew of their existence. It is excellent that the problem is not so severe or at its full strength yet and your body is taking care of it before it could turn into a serious illness. So if you realize the true cause of why you are feeling bad during fasting, your solution will be to continue with the fast. Your distress will quickly go away and you will feel just fine again. Continue your fast and win the fight with illnesses and aging.

Self-Testing by your Tongue.

Your tongue is a good indicator of what is going on inside of you and how you feel. If before your fast you completely cleansed your digestive system, than most likely your tongue came to its original, healthy, pink color. However, when you enter the fast, toxicity from other organs and cells is being dumped into your digestive system. Since your tongue is "a mirror" of your stomach, it shows you what is going on inside by covering up with the same residue. In the process of burning and flushing of toxicity from your digestive system, your tongue becomes clearer.

Depending on individuality and the level of toxic build up in the body, in order to completely cleanse your tongue, which means your whole system from toxicity- it is necessary to do 2-3 weeks fasting. In some cases that cycle needs to be repeated two or even three times with one month apart between the cycles. Clean, pink tongue after the fasting cycle indicates a completely cleansed system from toxicity and strong health.

Detailed Instructions
for Exiting the Fast

A Little Wisdom Please

During the fast, your body burned up a lot of old cells. When you start eating again, your body will use this new nutritional material to build new cells that were lost during fasting.

The question here is what level of quality do you want to have?

If you eat organic foods of the highest quality, you will build cells of the highest quality. If you chose to go back to eating processed foods with their burden of toxins built in, then you will get cells that come packaged with toxins. Why lose the ground you just gained?

Caveat Emptor

ATTENTION: The transition from fasting to regular food is very important. Breaking the rules of this transition period can undo all of the benefits and strengths of your fast. In fact, violating these rules can even harm your health.

On the other hand, strictly following these rules during this period will enhance the success of the cleansing therapy.

The Center is not responsible for any problems if you do not strictly abide by the rules found here.

> # The length of the
> # transition period
> # is equal to
> # the length of the fast.

STRICTLY PROHIBITED AFTER THE FAST

1. Don't use any SALT or any products containing salt.
2. Don't eat *fatty* or *spicy* foods.
3. Don't consume any milk or any milk products.
4. Don't use red meat, fish, chicken, turkey, etc.
5. Don't eat any canned foods.
6. Don't eat *dead foods*: foods that are not natural, that have been processed, that contain artificial ingredients, empty calories, are not fresh, have questionable quality, or are overcooked.
7. Don't eat to fullness. Overeating will produce toxins and make you feel weak and worse. (If you still feel hungry, you ate the right amount.)

STRICTLY EXPECTED PRACTICES FOR EXITING THE FAST

1. Do continue drinking vegetable and fruit juices (freshly made, natural, organic), herbal teas, and filtered water. (Fluids will decrease the feeling of hunger and compensate for the lesser amount of food.)

2. Do chew your food very thoroughly. This is important because chewing (and the mixing of saliva) is the first step in digestion. If an insufficient amount of saliva is mixed and/or food is not chewed thoroughly, then food does not digest fully. Incomplete digestion leads to toxins being formed in the body. This increases the work the digestive system must do, and therefore steals energy from the body.

3. Do continue with the procedures you used during fasting, such as dry-brush massage, walking, warm baths, jumping on rebounder, yoga, resting when tired, intentional relaxation, and light exercise with weights. Exercise with weights and yoga exercises will improve the circulation in muscles and in internal organs, promoting the building inside you of new, young, healthy cells.

4. After the first few days of fasting, the colon has so little in it for stimulation, that in order to keep it working, you will need to do Cleansing Exercises. Two times the first week, still do Colon Cleansing. During the second week, do a Colon Cleansing one time.

Exiting the Fast: A Schedule

First Day   You may skip some of this if you don't feel hungry.

7:00 a.m.   Drink 1 to 2 glasses of distilled water plus 1-2 tsp. strained lemon juice per glass.

9:00 a.m.   Drink the broth from cooked **brown** rice (1 or 2 tablespoons brown rice to 1 quart water.) Cook for about 40 minutes, then strain. *Find a place to sit undisturbed and think of something pleasant because this a very important time for your body, the moment of first food.* Drink the warm broth, **slowly.** Hold each sip in your mouth approximately 15 or 20 seconds. Drink one cup only.

> During this period, new cells are building from the food eaten and from the way this food is assimilated. So, to build up new, young and healthy cells, follow strictly all diet recommendations.

11:00 a.m.   Drink 1 cup warm herbal mint tea. (You may add 1 tsp. of strained lemon juice.)

1:00 p.m.   **Variation #1:** One clean, organic tomato blanched (dipped in boiling water for 10-15 seconds) and peeled; eat very slowly.

Variation #2: Five or six ounces of plain organic kefir.

3:00 p.m.   Drink one glass of any kind of vegetable juice (freshly made, natural, organic).

5:00 p.m.   **Variation #1:** One clean, organic, green, sour APPLE (*Granny Smith* variety), peeled, cored, shredded; eat very slowly.

Variation #2: Cooked brown rice soup (no more than 5 ounces, nothing more than rice, no salt, no sugar); eat very slowly; chew a minimum of 50 times.

7:00 p.m.   Drink vegetable broth, no more than 1 cup.

9:00 p.m.   Drink 1 cup camomile tea and 1 tsp. strained lemon juice.

Second Day

Persons who are underweight need to take a warm bath daily for the next one to two weeks, and, after the bath, lubricate the skin with warm olive oil, wait 20 minutes, and then take a warm shower.

Breakfast

Variation #1: 1 small whole, natural, organic, sour apple (Granny Smith), cleaned and peeled. (One more apple if desired.)

Variation #2: Whole oat soup: 3 tbs. oats, boiled in 1 quart water for 30 minutes or

156

more, until the oats are soft. Eat no more than 8 oz. or 200 grams, 1 glass.

Lunch   **Variation #1:** Finely shredded carrot (1 to 1 ½ medium carrots, 150 to 200 grams or 5-7 oz.).

Variation #2: Vegetable soup: Cut vegetables into small pieces; put them in already boiling water. Do not overcook; vegetables should still have a "crunch" to them when they are eaten. Do not eat more than 150 grams or 6 oz.

Dinner   **Variation #1:** Fresh salad (no more than 200 grams or 8 oz. or 1 cup):
Ingredients: shredded carrot, peeled and diced fresh cucumber, soft part of Romaine lettuce. Dressing: strained juice from lemon, no more than 1 tbs.

Variation #2: Whole oats, cooked until soft, eaten plain, no more than 100 grams or 5 to 6 oz. Don't add any dressing or seasoning.

Third Day With each meal, eat 1-2 average-sized cloves of garlic for the next 1 to 2 weeks.

Breakfast **Variation #1:** 1 sweet, fresh apple, 1 sweet pear, 250 to 300 grams or 10 oz.
Variation #2: 2 sweet apples.

Lunch   **Variation #1:** Whole brown rice, cooked

157

until soft, eaten plain, 100 to 150 grams or 5 to 7 oz. Don't add any dressing or seasoning.

Variation #2: Fresh salad (200 to 250 grams or 8 to 10 oz.) Ingredients: 1shredded carrot, ½ stick diced celery, ½ peeled and diced cucumber. Dressing: strained juice from fresh tomato.

Dinner **Variation #1:** Homemade vegetable soup, 150 to 200 grams or 8 to 10 oz.

Variation #2: Whole buckwheat or millet, cooked until soft, eaten plain, 100 to 150 grams or 5 to 7 oz. Don't add any dressing or seasoning.

Fourth Day

Breakfast Two fruits: either two sweet fruits or two sour fruits, but **not** sweet and sour combined. No more than 250 grams or 10 oz.

Lunch Fresh salad: four kinds of vegetables (carrot, cucumber, celery, lettuce, tomato) with sour dressing of lemon juice, grapefruit juice, or tomato juice.

Dinner Whole buckwheat plus steamed onions, carrots, and celery, cooked in their own juice. To steam vegetables in their own juice, add a small amount of water to the vegetables in a pan over low heat. The vegetables will

release their own juices for cooking. Eat no
more than 250 grams or 10 oz.

Fifth Day

Breakfast   Fruits of two or three kinds, but do not mix
sweet and sour fruits. No more than 250 to
300 grams or 10 to 12 oz.

Lunch   **Variation #1:** Vegetable soup plus one small,
steamed, organic potato. Do not eat more than
300 grams or 12 oz.

Variation #2: Fresh salad plus one small,
steamed, organic potato. Do not eat more
than 300 grams or 12 oz.

Dinner   Whole buckwheat or millet or oats or brown
rice or quinoa, plus onion, carrot, and celery,
cooked in their own juice. Just before eating
add 1 tsp. olive oil (organic, cold pressed,
virgin). Eat no more than 250 grams or 10 oz.

Days Six Through Fourteen (General Instructions)

Breakfast   Main food is fresh fruits or dried fruits,
soaked in water overnight.

Lunch   Fresh salad with steamed potato or any kind
of cooked grains.

Dinner   Vegetable soup, or any kind of grains with vegetables cooked in their own juice. During dinner, you may add to each serving 1 tbs. olive oil.

After two weeks, carefully add new foods: legumes (very well cooked), raw nuts, and sometimes a small amount of fish in correct combination, etc. *Good luck!*

Exiting the Fast with Transition to a Living Food Diet

If you want to go on a living food diet, fasting is the best way to start. Juice fasting in itself is a living food diet, therefore exiting the fast on raw food will be a logical continuation of this diet.

Caution: People who have weak digestion, bloating, and other stomach problems need to choose only those foods which agree with their digestion. When your digestion improves you can gradually introduce new foods and pay attention to how your digestion reacts.

If some food still creates discomfort, you should avoid that food now and try it again later if desired. Possibly during that time your digestion will improve, and then you will be able to eat that food. If not, if it again produces discomfort, indigestion, or gas, then wait.

Don't rush to get all of the vitamins and minerals possible at once. If you try to get the widest variety of food to get more nutrients when your digestion is not ready to handle the variety, instead of nutrients, you will get a large portion of toxins and toxic gases.

However, your body needs nutrition which may not be in the food you eat. Therefore, compensate for this lack of nutrients through fresh juices and liquid vitamins and minerals.

When you enter the fast with transition to the living food diet, follow the same rules as listed in the first part of this chapter.

Day 1

Breakfast   **Fruit Smoothie**

1. In Champion Juicer, make juice from oranges, grapefruit, apples, pineapples, or any two of these in combination.
2. Put pulp through the juicer 2-4 times to make juice thicker and more nutritional.
3. Pour juice into Vita-Mix and add pieces of mango or papaya.
4. Add 3-4 ice cubes made from pure water.
5. Blend 15-30 seconds.
6. If this is too sweet, squeeze some lemon juice into it.
7. Drink.
After breakfast, continue as on fast. Drink juices, herbal tea, and water.

Day 2

Breakfast   Same as Day One.

Lunch   **Vegetable Soup**

1. In Champion Juicer, make juice from carrots and celery.
2. Put pulp through the juicer 1-2 times to make juice thicker and more nutritional.
3. Pour juice into Vita-Mix and add pieces of tomato, cucumber, green pepper, or zucchini, or a combination of 2-3 of these. Juice should always cover the pieces.
4. Blend and drink.
Continue to drink juices, herbal tea, and water as on the fast.

Day 3

Breakfast   **Fruit Smoothie**
Same as Day One, but add to the Fruit Smoothie half a bunch of spinach in the blender.

Lunch   **Vegetable Soup**
Same as Day Two, but add to the Vegetable Soup some kale leaves in the blender.

Dinner   **Vegetable Juice**
In any vegetable juice add 1 tsp. flax seed oil. Between meals, drink water, herbal tea, and some juice.

Day 4

Breakfast   **Fruit Smoothie**
Same as Day Three, but add to the Fruit
Smoothie 1-2 Tbs. frozen fruits and 1 tsp.
flax seed oil in the blender.

Lunch   **Vegetable Soup**
Same as Day Three, but add to the Vegetable
Soup 1/3 ripe avocado and 1 medium-sized
clove of garlic in the blender.

Dinner   **Nut Milk**
1. Use 1-2 Tbs. soaked nuts: cashew, walnut,
or others. If almond, it is recommended to
peel the skin.
2. Put nuts into Vita-mix.
3. Add 1 c. apple juice and ½ c. pure water
   plus 3-4 pitted dates and 3-4 ice cubes.
4. Blend 60 seconds.
5. Strain and chew.

Day 5   Same as Day Four, but add 2 tsp. flax seed oil
for breakfast and ½ ripe avocado for lunch.

Day 6

Breakfast   **Fruit Salad**
Cut apples, kiwi, grapes, and put on a plate.
Pour over them the Fruit Smoothie made
from the recipe on Day Five.

Lunch   **Vegetable Soup**
Cut tomatoes, cucumber, some green onion
and bell pepper and pour over the Vegetable
Soup made from the recipe on Day Five.

Dinner   **Nut Milk**
Use 2-3 Tbs. nuts that have been soaked 8-12
hours. Blend, strain, and chew the same as on
Day Four.

Days 7-10

Continue the same as on Day Six.

Then you can carefully add other foods and pay
attention to the reaction of your digestion. Good luck!

Some Disorders and Illnesses Which Could Be Solved with Cell Cleansing

Chronic Fatigue, asthma, allergies, colds, skin problems, enlarged prostate, sexual disorders, digestive problems, weak immune system, insomnia, liver problems, fibroids, tumors, ...

SELF HELP: ___CELL CLEANSER___

Garlic/Lemon Tincture.
Take 4 lemons and 4 full garlic heads. Cut lemons in half and squeeze the juice out. Dice the peel in small pieces. Also use the seeds. Peel garlic and also dice. Put it in the glass jar and cover with 2.5 litters of water and keep for 5 days. Drink 2-4 oz per day until the solution is gone. Repeat the procedure every 3 months. This tincture cleanses blood vessels, liver and kidneys.

Other Important Services*

... at the Koyfman Center

This chapter will give an overview of cleansing services related to the eight steps described so far in this book. These services include:

- Weight Loss Cleansing Program

- Cleansing from Negative Emotions

- Stomach Cleansing

- Far Infrared Sauna

- Lung Cleansing

- Thyroid Cleansing Program

- Prostate Cleansing Program

- Urine Therapy

- Sinus Cleansing

Weight Loss
Cleansing Program

When properly and thoughtfully followed, this weight loss program will help you to lose unwanted and unhealthy weight without drugs or other chemicals and their unwelcome side effects. The weight loss program discussed here is not a "diet," and therefore avoids the inconsistent and sometimes harmful results that come from what is often hawked on television, etc.

How Many Pounds Do Toxins Weigh?

Many weight loss programs focus on losing excess fat. To accomplish this, they suggest various methods to burn fat, such as:

- intensive exercise without medical control (overweight people often have heart problems),
- pills which allow you to "eat everything and not gain weight,"
- pills which suppress your appetite, and
- fat-free diets where fats are artificially removed from foods making them more dangerous than the fat itself.

These methods play on only one aspect of losing fat, and then push that one aspect to the extreme. For example, some methods use excessive exercise without taking nutrition into account properly. Others starve the body by the use of chemicals that suppress the appetite. (Some of these hunger suppressing pharmaceuticals are not far removed from some illegal street drugs.) The list goes on.

These unbalanced techniques are too often dangerous. Sometimes (rarely) people have died from these diets or programs. More often their health suffers because after they finish losing the desired weight, they go back to the same old habits that caused them to be overweight in the first place. They regain the lost weight rapidly, and this "whiplashes" the body. This does more harm to both physical and emotional health than the temporary benefits of weight loss.

Worst of all, these artificial weight loss programs ignore a very simple but vital fact: There are two different types of excess weight: excess fat and toxic weight.

A very significant percentage of excess weight in the average person living in the industrialized world is not fat at all; it is toxic weight. This weight accumulates in the internal organs such as the large intestine, the liver, the kidneys, the lymph glands, the small intestine, joints and the stomach. These wastes come packaged in many forms with various compositions. They include colon stones, toxic mucus, liver and gall stones, toxic bile, kidney stones, toxic lymph fluids, and uric acids, to name a few.

As if this were not bad enough, add to this toxic brew the weight and wastes of parasites. Some modern people scoff at the notion that they could have parasites, but the overwhelming evidence, and the indisputable testimonies of the highest ranking national medical professionals make it clear that this is not strictly a phenomenon of Third World countries. It is prevalent here in the United States. (See the chapter on Parasite Cleansing in my book, *Deep Internal Body Cleansing.*)

Parasites thrive on toxins accumulated in the body. After eating such toxins, they excrete new, even more dangerous toxins and gases. For some people these gases accumulate in tissues and can make a person feel and look bloated.

While it is true that excess fat is bad for your health, toxic weight (and parasites) pose a worse problem in terms of excess weight. For example, on the walls of the large intestine alone anywhere from 20-70 pounds of toxic weight can accumulate. This is the weight we need to get rid of first. Additionally, toxic weight which accumulates on the walls of our organs and cells is weight which provides the foundation of disease.

When you get rid of the weight of toxins, you get rid of the weight of your diseases.

What Organs Do We Need to Cleanse to Get Rid of Toxic Weight?

Toxins come into the human system in several different ways, through breathing (inhalation), through eating and drinking (ingestion), and through the skin (absorption). Rarely do toxins enter through injection. Of these different pathways into the body, the most likely route is an improper diet.

Each organ is affected differently, depending on the toxins, the route of entry, and the diverse chemistry in the individual body. Regardless of individual differences, the fact remains that toxic weight accumulates in the organs of our bodies. Which organ is affected more than another depends on personal circumstances.

The colon (large intestine) is the main sewer of the body, and logically accumulates the largest amount of toxic weight. The other digestive organs, the stomach, and the small intestine, are also impacted.

It is also easily understood that the organs that filter out chemical and microscopic biological toxins (the liver and the kidneys) are also heavily contaminated. Like any other filter, they become clogged with time and usage. As they do their work, toxic weight builds up in these critical organs.

The lungs and sinuses are in direct contact with our polluted environment. As such they get "dosed" with airborne contaminants ranging from dust mites, to chemicals from sprays, to vehicle exhaust, to bacteria and viruses. These can physically clog the respiratory system or cause allergic reactions (allergies).

Toxic weight can also be found on the walls of blood vessels, in lymph and lymph nodes, in the pancreas, and in each cell.

Cleansing Leads to Weight Loss, Which Leads to Healing

Deep body cleansing, along with following the principles of healthy eating and a healthy lifestyle, not only lead to losing weight, but also help to heal the body from disease and to rejuvenate the body. This is because, as toxins are cleansed from the body, the metabolism normalizes and helps the body to burn fat the way it is supposed to.

How Much Time Will It Take to Lose Weight Through Cleansing?

On an average, losing weight through "modern" diets takes an advertised 30 days. Unfortunately, in even less time your weight comes back even more than it was before. In addition, there could be new health problems.

On the other hand, losing weight through deep internal body cleansing, as described in this book, does take longer. The difference is that its moderate speed helps to make it safer and longer lasting. The fact that this kind of natural weight loss is really a lifestyle and not a fad means that you will keep the excess fat off for as long as you maintain the lifestyle.

Just as each organ in your body is different in size, shape, and weight, so the cleansing of each of these different organs removes differing amounts and types of toxic weight. You lose the most toxic weight when you cleanse the colon, lymph, liver, and cells.

The very best results come from a combination of cleansing, eating a "living food" diet, and exercise. For 2-6 months, you may lose from 30-100 pounds of toxic weight cleansed from the internal organs as well as "toxic fat." With such an approach you not only lose weight, you look better, have more energy, and in general feel yourself re-born. **Notice:** With such a method of losing weight, the skin regains its shape and elasticity, leaving no wrinkles from being overweight.

Recommended Diet during the Weight Loss program or for Maintenance

Simple Raw Food Recipes:

These recipes can be used during "fasting" from cooked foods, as well as on regular daily basis. During that "fast" the amount of food you eat in one meal should not exceed 200-300grams (8-12oz). The food has to be eaten very slow chewing every bit very well. It is better if you eat only two times per day. The rest of the time, you may drink fresh juices, herbal tea (without sugar), water and vegetable broth. This regiment will support your energy, satisfy your hunger and allow you to lose extra pounds.

Breakfast Options:

1. Apples, papaya and ½ avocado blended into puree.
2. A Melon.
3. Any favorite fruit in season (not more than 2-3 types mixed together).

Dinner Options:

- One banana + ½-1 cups of grapes blended. Add 5-7 cubes of ice. Instead of banana, you may use mango or papaya. (Those have problems with yeast, this blend is not recommended).
- Romaine Lettuce (one bunch) with 5 presoaked dates and 5-7 walnuts (soaked and dried).
- Two carrots with 1-2 cloves of garlic + ½ avocado. Put everything in the food processor to mix it up.

Instead of avocado you may use 1-2 table spoons of organic sour cream.

Please look for more recipes in my book *"Healing Through Cleansing Diet"*.

It is recommended to follow this diet from one week to one month.

The goals of this type of diet are:

- Weight loss
- Rest for digestive organs
- Feeding the system with enzymes, vitamins, minerals and other life and vital elements.

Therapeutic Benefits of Weight Loss with the Cleansing Method

- Eliminates unpleasant smells from skin (You don't need to use deodorant any more.)
- Improves skin and skin color
- Better sleep
- Improves concentration
- More energy and stamina
- Normalizes blood pressure
- Eliminates pain from joints and back
- Improves vision
- Increases flexibility
- Increases clarity of the mind (Some have said the mind works like a computer after this cleansing.)
- During 6-10 months of cleansing procedures and healthy lifestyle, you can look 10-15 years younger.

Cleansing from
Negative Emotions

Cleansing your body, mind, heart, soul, and spirit from negative emotions will provide a surprising boost to the other cleansings, and to overall health status.

Cleansing Number One

Cleansing the body from negative emotions is one of the most important cleansings. In many cases, without this cleansing other cleansing procedures give only temporary results.

Because negative emotions accumulate not only in the physical body (organs, muscles, blood vessels, nerves, and other tissues) but also in the energy field, we need to do cleansing on all levels.

In our Center we start cleansing from negative emotions with physical cleansing procedures. Such an approach gives quick improvement of general conditions and the client becomes more capable of doing other methods of cleansing from negative emotions by himself or herself.

How Negative Thoughts and Emotions Affect the Body

Frequently repeated negative thoughts and emotions can cause tension in muscles and organs so that they tighten up like a frightened animal trying to hide from danger. After the stress has passed, these tensions do not completely disappear but leave behind a "residue" of stress. Unfortunately, these residues can build up with each significant incident.

Problems from this build-up of tension take several different forms. For example, the tension in muscles and organs uses up some of the energy of the body, weakening its immune system. This constant but low-grade tension also contributes to blockages that hinder the circulation of nutrients, blood, lymph, oxygen, energy, etc.

Stress from negative emotions promotes an increased secretion of hormones into the blood. In natural stress situations, such as "fight or flight" physical danger, a person uses up these hormones through increased physical activity such as running, fighting, or working. These hormones are burned up by the muscles, and do not cause harm.

However, in today's social settings, negative emotions are usually not acted upon physically. Therefore, your anger stays inside of you. The large amounts of hormones secreted— instead of being burned off by muscles or used in digestion— attack and harm various organs.

Suppressed or unrealized emotions are the reason for the unbalance in different organs.

More information about negative emotions and cleansing the body from them can be read in Books 2 and 3 of my series, *Healing through Cleansing,* and in my book, *Deep Internal Body Cleansing.*

Cleansing Method to Eliminate Negative Emotions

- Stomach Cleansing
- Complex Liver Cleansing
- Small Intestine Cleansing
- Fasting

Therapeutic Benefits of Cleansing from Negative Emotions

- Eliminate fear, anger, jealousy, etc.
- Make you calm, relaxed, and peaceful.
- Make you balanced.
- Give you more confidence.
- Make you feel secure.
- Make you think positively.
- Give you feelings of hope.
- Make you feel happy.
- Improve your defense against diseases.

Stomach
Cleansing

The Importance of Stomach Cleansing to Your Health

The stomach is that very important organ where either good health or bad health begins.

This is true because the stomach begins the digestive process where your food is separated into nutrients your body needs and waste materials that carry toxins.

Over time, the waste that is not properly removed from the body will stick to the walls of the digestive tract. These wastes build up, thin layer upon thin layer just like plaque in the arteries. Gradually, these layers thicken and create a perfect environment in which disease bacteria, parasites and other unhealthy micro-organisms can thrive.

If this waste lining is not periodically removed it will also interfere with the *production* of digestive juices, and the proper *mixing* of these gastric juices with the chyme.

Poor eating habits are to blame for a variety of stomach problems. Some of those poor eating habits include the following:

1. *Overeating* causes food to ferment in the stomach.
2. *Improper food combinations* cause incomplete digestion, thereby creating excess waste.
3. *Eating "fast foods"* introduces chemical additives which poison the body.

4.   *Eating before going to sleep* stresses the entire digestive system. Your body is supposed to be at rest, yet because of food in the stomach, it has to work during sleep. Digestion takes a lot of energy.

As a result of these unfortunate conditions, the body wastes precious disease-fighting energy in inefficient, poorly timed digestion, and on fighting the unwelcome micro-organisms that grow in the uncleansed digestive tract. This can lead to symptoms ranging from acid indigestion and acid reflux, to constipation, gastritis, and ulcers, plus diseases such as cancer.

There are 24,000 new cases of stomach cancer in the United States each year. Although the cause for stomach cancer is not certain, there is an association with gastritis.

One cause of ulcers and gastritis are infections from the recently discovered bacterium *Heliobacter pylori*. Such micro-organisms cannot live in clean, healthy stomachs. Therefore, it is essential that the stomach be kept cleansed to keep this and other bacteria from growing.

Critical to your personal health is the fact that the stomach provides nutrients to the different organs of the immune system. It also supports the good bacteria that inhabit the colon, and controls the proper elimination of wastes. Therefore, good nutrition combined with cleansing the digestive system are vital to developing and then preserving good health.

In order to remove these problems, regular cleansing of the stomach is needed. Stomach Cleansing uses natural methods, gently and safely, to cause the stomach to release these long-term, accumulated wastes for elimination. This procedure removes the environment required by parasites and harmful micro-organisms. With these unwelcome life forms gone, the immune system no longer needs to fight them.

By removing stored wastes, Stomach Cleansing removes poisonous chemicals and harmful bacteria (toxins) that are an additional burden to the immune system. This permits the immune system to fight diseases and invading bacteria with greater strength and effectiveness.

Stomach Cleansing is one technique used as part of the program of "Deep Internal Body Cleansing." Using herbs, organic juices and massage, "Deep Internal Body Cleansing" can cause the body to release wastes that poison the immune system and interfere with its ability to heal itself.

This procedure can only be properly accomplished by trained, experienced professionals who understand these techniques. Koyfman Whole Body Cleansing has more than a half century of professional experience in "Deep Internal Body Cleansing" techniques that help the body flush away wastes and heal itself. The Center has both up-to-date equipment and international experience that together provide the maximum in internal cleansing.

Benefits

- Enhances your digestion.
- Activates function of the pancreatic glands and liver.
- Cleanses the stomach from stagnated bile.
- Purges mucus from the bronchus and lungs.
- Helps lessen the symptoms of allergies, nasal congestion, colds, flu, etc.
- Expels poisonous matter from the stomach through a powerful technique.
- Improves mood, emotions, and outlook on life.
- Calms the nerves and spirit.

Description of Technique

This cleansing is recommended for those who have a good "vomiting reflex." If you don't have a strong "gag reflex," we suggest that you substitute a Whole Digestive System Cleansing followed by a Small Intestine Cleansing. Materials to have on hand include a tub of several gallon size capacity, paper towels or napkins, and a wet face cloth.

1. Cleansing of the upper stomach (that bulbous part that first receives food) must be done only on an empty stomach, and preferably in the morning after toiletries and morning exercises. (If necessary, this procedure can be done at any time as long as the stomach is empty.)

2. First drink two or three glasses of the solution provided. Drink it in the kitchen or in the restroom while either sitting or squatting comfortably. Make sure your spine is straight while drinking the solution. Sit in a straight-backed chair or stand or walk. If you bend forward while drinking you squeeze the stomach. The speed of drinking should be rather fast, a cup every 1-2 minutes, in order to lessen absorption. (The virtue of this solution is not in being absorbed as if it were food.)

3. Throughout the procedure, do the steps calmly and deliberately. It is important not to strain or stretch your muscles.

- Wash your hands thoroughly
- Position yourself near the tub.
- Wet two fingers in clean warm water but do not wipe them dry. Leave them wet.
- Close your eyes, and put the other hand on your stomach. Make a fist with that other hand and press inward and upward on the upper abdomen to help the stomach release its contents.
- Take a deep, slow breath.
- Put the two wet fingers down your throat and press down on the root of the tongue to stimulate the "gag reflex."
- Bend slightly over the tub, exhale, and then vomit a small amount in one or two cycles. **Do this gently.**
- **Note:** This is not the same as nausea. This is a highly controlled activity or movement. It is done from the mind, and with the same precision as an exercise. Think in terms of simply emptying the contents of the stomach. Because your stomach is empty except for the solution, the sensation will not be anywhere near as unpleasant as vomiting partially digested food.

Caution: Do not try to empty the stomach 100% because that can stress the heart or cause you to feel discomfort and tiredness.

- Take long, deep breaths through your mouth by inhaling gently along the two fingers still inserted in your mouth. (Be careful not to gulp or gasp air.) Deep, slow breathing is important.
- After one vomiting cycle, clean your fingers, mouth, face, and nose with running water under the faucet, with a paper towel, or with a cool, wet face cloth previously placed within reach.

4. Drink two or three more glasses of solution.

5. Repeat again one or two cycles of vomiting.

6. Drink two to four more glasses of solution.

7. Try to vomit with more strength and volume, while being careful not to stress yourself too much.

8. Take a 30 to 60 second break between cycles.

    "Divided Drinking" is a technique of drinking the warm water solution in stages, not all at once. This technique is beneficial because with every repeated cycle of "divided drinking," the vomiting becomes easier. This is a benefit not found by drinking the solution all at once and regurgitating it all at once. Another benefit of "divided drinking" is that by not filling the stomach to the limit, you prevent that over-full feeling, and you do not stress the heart.

9. The final period of cleansing comes when all of the solution has been drunk. **This period is very**

important. During this time, without drinking, try to empty the stomach as much as possible, making the rest of the solution come up. Divide this final period into cycles, taking breaks between cycles. Breaks should last 30 seconds in the beginning, then increase to one minute then to three minutes and more. This gives you more rest, and a better opportunity to listen to your body to find the best moment to vomit. Continue to vomit until you sense the bitter taste, see the yellow color of bile, and feel the burping stop. Finish when you feel calm and empty inside.

10. To bring your stomach to a balanced, normal condition in which it feels calm and relaxed, drink one-half glass of cool, pure water, or an herbal tea. This tea can be made from camomile, but without honey. Then take a warm shower, lie down, and relax. Even though the entire procedure must take about one hour, the active cleansing will take 20 to 30 minutes.

11. Do not eat anything for a minimum of three hours after completing this procedure. Let this organ rest.

12. If you are experiencing any stomach problems, eat well-cooked brown rice or buckwheat with butter, but no sooner than three hours after the procedure. This tends to settle the stomach.

13. If you are not having stomach problems, (usually the case) you may eat vegetarian meals.

14. It is better to learn this procedure under professional supervision. After you become proficient in it

yourself, you should consider repeating this procedure about every two to four weeks for maintenance purposes.

15.   If you do not practice good eating habits, and/or if you have a candida overgrowth, it may be necessary to do this procedure more often.

Signs of Candida Overgrowth

1.   The urine is not clear, possibly with bubbles and foam.
2.   Feces float because the gasses produced by candida are mixed with the feces.
3.   Discomfort in the stomach, or in the abdomen area (excessive burping, bloating, gas, etc.).

(You can find other symptoms in Donna Gates' book, *The Body Ecology Diet*.)

How to Make the Solution

Take 1-3 quarts of clean purified water, and warm it to body temperature. (Do not use a microwave oven for this.) Add 1 teaspoon of sea salt per 1 quart of water and mix thoroughly.

Caution: Do not do this procedure if you have high blood pressure or a serious heart problem. In this case, do an easier variation of Stomach Cleansing which is described in my book, *Healing Through Cleansing*, Book 3. Also use this alternative technique if you don't have a natural gag reflex.

Some Disorders and Illnesses Which Could Be Solved with Stomach Cleansing

Weak digestion, nausea, headache, sinus problems, burping, sore throat, colds, flu, coughing, asthma, allergies.

Testimonial:

"...I have been coughing horribly all the time for over 10 years. It caused by the chemical fumes I have worked with all my life. I thought it was hopeless and I'd never be cured from that discomfort. When I came to Dr. Koyfman, he recommended some dietary changes and cleansing procedures. He was ver knowledgeable and it was easy to trust him. At first stomach cleansing scared me, but it turned out to be very easy, gentle and most importantly effective. After my first stomach cleansing, I did not cough for 2 days. It was amazing! When the cough did come back, it wasn't as strong and as often. After few more visits, I am cough free!..."   *Donna R.*

SELF HELP: <u>*STOMACH ULCERS*</u>

If you have stomach ulcers:
1. Drink freshly made carrot (200 grams)+ cabbage (50gr.) Juice 3 times per day, 30 minutes before meals. Juice needs to be drunk immediately after making.

2. Mix 1 tablespoon of rye-bran in 8 oz of warm water. Drink in small sips 30 minutes before each meal for 3-6 months.

Self-Testing
During the Stomach Cleansing

Reasons of Indigestion and Stomach disorders.

As it was mentioned before, on the walls of the stomach accumulate mucus, leftovers of undigested foods, which start to ferment and rot, producing a very unpleasant smell, which can often be noticed from the mouth. On the bottom of the stomach can often be found toxic bile. That bile gets into the stomach if a person eats late at night, overeats or combines foods improperly. Due to that, functioning of the valve, which connects stomach and the small intestine, impairs and it is not able to close completely. Through that slightly open valve, bile from the liver and small intestine gets into the stomach and settles on the bottom of it. Accumulation of that toxic bile causes different disorders, such as Acid Reflux, Heart Burn, etc.

Mucus and undigested foods create a wonderful environment for bacteria, infection, viruses and other parasites. These creatures can cause different stomach illnesses, such as gastritis, ulcers and even cancer. For instance H-Pylori is a widespread bacteria, which causes gastric ulcers and if not treated properly and in timely manner, can cause cancer.

Stress, negative emotions and depression can lead to stomach problems as well. Negative emotions create tension in the stomach muscles, which causes digestive glands to produce less digestive juices and worsen digestion. These tension spots become a perfect home for toxicity and bad bacteria for reproduction.

What can you see?

To see better what comes out of your stomach during the Stomach Cleansing procedure, you have to release its contents into a bucket or large bowl. After stomach cleanse, you can see chunks of mucus, undigested food, foam, bubbles, yeast and sometimes other parasites. You may also taste a horrible sourness or bitterness in the mouth. Even if it seem that the "water" released from your stomach is clean and it does not have anything abnormal, be brave and feel it with your hand. You will feel a gooey, sticky, heavy, glue-like substance. That glue-like substance covers the stomach walls damaging functioning of digestive glands. It becomes an excellent feeding ground for unfriendly bacteria and infection. So indigestion, burping, headaches and other disorders mentioned earlier, are the result a result of that toxic layer.

What illnesses are caused by stomach toxicity?

Besides that toxicity weakening stomach's functioning, causing its illnesses, it also absorbs into blood and spreads into other organs causing sinuses, headaches, ear infections, eye problems, colds, soar throat, pneumonia, allergies, etc. That is why regular cleansing of the stomach is good to prevent these illnesses. If these illnesses are already present, stomach cleansing will drastically help improve the way you feel. By combining cleansing with a healthy life style, healthy eating and regular exercise, can help you get rid of these problems completely.

How quickly do stomach walls clog back up after stomach cleansing procedure?

If you are one of very few people who have a perfect diet, absolutely no stress, regular exercise routine, get outside fresh air daily for prolonged time– then congestion of the stomach walls is much slower. For these individuals, stomach cleansing with change of season, once per three months, could be enough. In individuals who are not able to follow all principles of healthy eating, rarely spend time outside, do not exercise regularly– stomach walls clog up much faster. So in that case, in order to prevent stomach problems and connected organs, it is necessary to do a stomach cleanse once per month. Those who do not follow any rules of healthy eating, do not exercise and are constantly under stress and accumulate mucus easily, should do stomach cleansing more often- two to four times per month or ideally once per week.

How can you find out if you have a predisposition for a quick mucus accumulation?

If you often have colds, sinuses, clogged nose, throat problems, allergies and headaches, regularly cough up mucus (especially in the morning after awakening)– you are definitely a person who quickly accumulates mucus.
Regular stomach cleansing will help you remove mucus and prevent occurrence of many illnesses.

Far Infrared Sauna

    Far Infrared heat produces rays, which warm the body to the cellular level. In the Far Infrared Sauna, you sweat 2-3 times more than in regular saunas. One can actually burn from 300 to 600 and sometimes up to 900 calories per session! Also, during the session we serve hot cleansing tea and fresh squeezed juice. You feel comfortable and relaxed!

    Even in ancient times - for example the Roman Empire - people have used saunas not only to relax the mind and the body, but to heal the body of various ailments. This pleasant, relaxing technique has been used in numerous cultures across the planet for the past two millennia to provide health benefits that are not easily duplicated otherwise.

Therapeutic Benefits of Cleansing FIR-Sauna Include:

- Weight Loss
- Cleansing from Heavy Metals
- Cleansing of Thyroid Gland
- Activation of blood and lymph system circulation
- Cleansing of blood vessels
- Cleansing of lymph glands
- Help in fighting colds, flu and other infections
- Cleansing of muscle tissue
- Cleansing of the skin
- Helping the skin to better able to "breathe"
- Decrease the demand on the lungs and kidneys
- Decrease the general level of toxins in the body

▸ Activation of internal organ

Please note that those organs, glands and body parts where more sweat is produced, cleanse better!

How Does a Cleansing Sauna Work?

While in the heated environment of the sauna, the body's temperature is raised to a carefully pre-set level to cause all of the organs in the body to release toxins to the skin. As the heat causes the body to perspire, the toxins are flushed from the body in the sweat. This is a natural method of causing your body to give up wastes it has been storing for many years.

Herbal Teas and Natural Juices

While you are in the sauna, you will enjoy a herbal tea that the staff will provide to you. After this, freshly made vegetable juices will also be provided for you to drink. Both of these beverages are designed to stimulate your organs and systems to gently release toxins your body has stored for years.

The herbal teas and natural juices work in harmony with the heat of the sauna to maximize the purging or cleansing effect of the sauna. While you are calmly sitting back drinking herbal teas and organic juices your body is flushing toxins from your body to clear the way for you to better health.

What Specific Benefits Should I Expect to Receive From a Cleansing Sauna?

The cleansing sauna enlists the aid of the body's largest elimination organ, the skin, to release toxins through the pores.

Who Needs a Cleansing Sauna?

A cleansing sauna is like taking a shower from the inside out. This is important because the processed food we eat and the often unclean air we breathe brings into our bodies toxic materials that slowly accumulate over time. A cleansing sauna opens up channels in the body it needs to flush these toxins out. Internal cleansing is often as important as external cleansing.

Testimonial:

"...This is like science fiction! I came to the center knowing I had a heavy metal problem. I have tried many different ways to get rid of it, but everything seemed helpless. Dr. Koyfman recommended different cleanses including FIR Sauna. I have tried it before as well, but it was not as effective as doing it in combination with colon cleansing. Dr. Koyfman also has a good method of giving special herbal tea and a fresh juice. After I finished my sauna, I noticed that the towel I was sitting on has silver coloring on it. It scared me, but Dr. Koyfman explained that those were actual heavy metals which came out with my sweat..."

Brian D.

Self- Testing
During FIR-Sauna

So how are toxins being released while you are in the FIR-Sauna?

If done in our center, warming-up and dissolution of toxicity in the sauna, happens through three channels.

1. The main warming happens through irradiation of infrared rays, which penetrate deep into the organs and cells. This process expands all pathways and blood vessels, dissolves toxicity so it becomes runnier and more movable. Pores of the skin also expand and open-up letting the dissolved toxicity to come out through sweating.

2. In the sauna, you begin drinking hot tea made out of cleansing herbs. The tea will activate liver and kidney functions. The hot water will warm-up the stomach. If the stomach is warmed, it warms-up close by organs: liver, pancreas, spleen, and upper parts of the colon and small intestine. From the stomach hot water quickly absorbs into the bloodstream. The blood also warms-up and much better dissolves toxicity stuck to the walls of blood vessels. Taking in consideration that is not just water, but cleansing herbs, and that the blood vessels and capillaries go through all organs and glands of internal secretion, you can understand that this cleansing process includes the whole body.
    After you drink your hot tea, we give you a freshly squeezed fruit or vegetable juice, which also has

cleansing and activation powers. Alive vitamins, minerals, enzymes and electro-lights quickly absorb into the blood, which caries them through all body organs feeding them and activating their functions. In addition, it activates organs and cells stimulating cleansing.

3.   Third level of warming-up happens through the lungs, by deeper and slower breathing. Hot air travels through the nose pathways, sinuses, bronchis and gets into the lungs. By traveling through all those channels, hot air dissolves accumulated in those organs toxicity and mucus, killing infections as well. In addition, by getting in the lungs, hot air warms-up the lungs, and through them other organs–heart, stomach, diaphragm, etc. In the lungs, hot oxygen is absorbed by blood and warms it as well.

How do you determine where the cleansing by the sauna is more active?

Although cleansing of the whole body occurs, while in the sauna you can easily determine which organs, glands and parts of the body are cleansing the most. When you can actually see for yourself which organ is cleansing, you psychologically add on to the physical cleansing process an element of convincement and assurance that the cleansing is effective.

So you may determine which organ or body part is cleansing the best- by noticing where you sweat the most. You can also find out how good the cleansing is going by intensity of sweating in that certain area. For instance:

If your **neck** is intensively sweating– it means that your tonsils and thyroid gland are cleansing from toxicity and heavy metals, preventing throat illnesses and disorders. Also are being cleansed blood vessels of the neck, which are connected to the brain and other vital organs. Improves circulation and function of the brain (memory, thinking, control of other organs) as well.

If your **lower back** is sweating– it means that not only skin and muscles of that area are being cleansed, but also all near by organs: kidneys and adrenal glands; spine from salts and uric acid; also improves flexibility. FIR-Sauna eases kidneys work load by removing excess water from the tissue, fatty cells, swollen joints and organs. By doing so it also eases the work of heart which constantly, day and night, has to circulate excess water (in the blood) throughout the body. You also loose toxic weight by removing excess water, which is not naturally removed because of the overwhelmed and tired kidneys.

If you notice sweating **under arms, on the chest and around solar plexis**– it means the main lymph nodes (filters of the lymphatic system) are being cleansed. Cleansing of the lymphatic system and lymph nodes prevents breast cysts/tumors and lymphatic illnesses.

Sweating in the **abdominal area** means cleansing of liquid substances of digestive organs and the space between them. Reproductive organs located in that area are being cleansed as well. Etc...

FIR-Sauna is a powerful tool to cleanse blood vessels, blood, lymphatic system, thyroid gland, kidneys, sinuses, skin, muscle and tissue cells as well as dissolution of fatty cells. This amazing procedure,

- ▸ Dissolves and evacuates toxic mucus, heavy metals and chemical elements accumulated in the blood vessels, lymph and even cells of the body.
- ▸ Kills bad bacteria and infection in the sinuses, bronchis and lungs.

- Heals and Prevents different types of colds.
- Activates circulation.
- Burns extra calories.
- Helps to loose toxic weight (the weight of all your illnesses).
- Relaxes stress tensions.
- Improves your mood.

* Self testing in the Sauna will help you understand the effectiveness of this pleasurable as well as beneficial cleansing procedure.

Testimonials:

"...FIR Sauna is so much different from the regular sauna. I never felt good after being in the regular dry heat. After the Sauna in the Koyfman Center with their unique technique, special tea and freshly squeezed juice, I felt great! My pores opened up. The skin felt smooth. I felt relaxed and energized for the rest of the day. I also noticed that having the FIR Sauna in combination with other cleansing procedures is very effective..."

Jim D.

"...together with other cleanses, FIR Sauna worked great for my skin. It used to look so toxic, but now my pores are open, pimples and other impurities are gone. I am actually able to sweat again. It feels good to be able to lose toxins through the skin and sweat."

Marsha K.

Lung
Cleansing

Weak Lungs - Poor Health

Of all of the "nutrients" that we need for life, air is the most important because its absence will kill you sooner than an absence of food or water. The lungs are also important for nourishing and cleansing the blood cells and all the organs.

Lungs can be weakened by such things as toxic mucus, tobacco residues, airborne chemicals, bacteria and viruses, and a host of other contaminants. The success of any cleansing offered by the Center may well rest upon the health of the lungs.

Lung Cleansing includes cleansing not only the lungs themselves but also the entire air passageway which leads to the lungs: the branchiae, sinuses, and nasal passages.

Who Needs Lung Cleansing?

Practically everybody needs Lung Cleansing and the improvement of lung function, especially
- People who work in unclean air with chemicals, spray paint, and other sprays
- Those who smoke now or did so previously
- Those who have poor digestion
- Those who frequently catch colds and flu

- Those who have allergies, asthma
- Those who have a weak heart
- Those who have depression, frequent stress, weak immune systems and chronic fatigue.

What Is Lung Cleansing?

In my system any cleansing procedure consists of two parts. One part is the part you do yourself described in the series of four books, *Healing through Cleansing*. I recommend these books to everybody who is interested in improving his or her health.

The second part is the part you do at our Center with professional help. Lung Cleansing in our center includes cleansing the whole digestive system which is the main channel by which to eliminate toxins from the body because the digestive system has connections with all other parts of the body.

During the cleansing we utilize techniques which dilute toxins in the lungs, branchiae, and sinuses, and then pull them to the stomach. From the stomach they go to the small intestine, then to the colon and then out.

Notice: *The client receives more detailed information about Lung Cleansing during the individual consultation in our Center.*

Cleansing the lungs is a simple procedure which yields a great result.

Therapeutic Benefits of Lung Cleansing

- Greater immunity to colds and allergies
- Improved digestion
- Increased oxygen nourishment for cells and organs
- Improved blood quality
- Reduced amount of toxins in the body
- Heart function strengthened
- Normalized blood pressure
- Nervous system relaxed and calmed

Short List of Disorders Which Could Be Helped with this Cleansing

- Asthma
- Colds
- Sinus Problems
- Allergies
- Depression
- Digestive Disorders
- Sleep Disorders
- Heart Problems
- Breathing Difficulties
- Weakened Immune System

Thyroid Cleansing Program

The thyroid gland is so small it is often overlooked in considering one's personal health program. The Koyfman Center Thyroid Cleansing Program gives this gland its due place.

King of Glands

The thyroid gland is a little butterfly-shaped organ at the base of the neck that puts out a teaspoon of hormone a year. This hormone affects the metabolism and acts as cellular carburetor for every cell in the body—from the hair follicles down to the toenails.

If the thyroid gland is functioning properly, it acts as a fortress which defends our bodies from the invasion of illness. If the function of the thyroid gland is abnormal or impaired, it can lead to a variety of emotional and physical disorders.

What Is the Reason for Thyroid Gland Impairment?

Each organ and gland receives its nutrients from the blood.

If the liver is overloaded with toxins it will not be able to cleanse the blood, and toxins or poisons will spread throughout the body via the blood vessels and lymph. In this case the thyroid gland gradually accumulates toxins on its surface. As these toxic deposits thicken, they eventually block the path by which the thyroid gland receives nutrients.

Iodine is the number one nutrient for the thyroid gland. If the fluids we drink and the foods we eat don't have enough of this mineral, the function of the thyroid gland can become impaired.

What Health Problems Can Be Caused by an Impaired Thyroid Gland?

- Weakness
- Dry Coarse Skin
- Slow Speech
- Coarse Hair
- Hair Loss
- Weight Gain
- Difficulty Breathing
- Problems with Menstruation
- Nervousness
- Heart Palpitations
- Severe Chronic Fatigue
- Depression

When the thyroid isn't working properly, the immune system is impaired and this sets up a vicious cycle.

"...For seventeen years I have been on thyroid medication. But even with the medication I was overweight, my metabolism was slow and I had a chronic fatigue. When I came to Dr. Koyfman, he explained the whole concept behind the thyroid malfunctioning and suggested a program. After only a few cleanses I felt a big difference, but after my third Liver Cleanse, I stopped my medication completely. For maintenance, I follow Dr. Koyfman's recommendations and diet. I am amazed that the result is staying with me, it is not a short term thing..."   *Leslie K.*

How the Thyroid Function can be Restored

To cleanse the thyroid gland one must first lay a very powerful foundation.

- Cleanse the whole digestive system. This is a foundational procedure to open the main channel to eliminate toxins and stop their spreading.
- Completely cleanse the liver.
- Cleanse the blood and lymph systems.
- Begin to eat healthfully, using green fresh juices which dilute toxins in the thyroid gland.
- Do exercises which activate circulation and restore function in the thyroid gland.

Notice: Diet, exercise, and special thyroid massage are described in Book 2 of my series, *Healing through Cleansing.*

Therapeutic Benefits of Thyroid Cleansing

- Sense of Strength
- Soft, Smooth Skin
- Improved Speech Patterns
- Healthy, Flowing Hair
- Possible Thickening of Hair
- Stabilized Weight
- Efficient Breathing
- Ease in Menstruation
- Calmness
- Heart Regularity and Rhythm
- More Energy
- Sense of Well Being and Hope

Prostate
Cleansing Program

Prostate Cleansing at the Koyfman Center may be your ticket to refreshing relief and pleasant results.

The prostate gland, located just below the bladder, is approximately the size of a walnut. It wraps around the urethra. The prostate generates seminal fluid, which is essential for the survival of sperm. This important gland also lubricates the urethra to prevent infection and promote sperm flow.

Main Reason for Prostate Dysfunction

All blood vessels and lymphatic fluids provide nutrition and normal functions for the prostate, testicles, penis and all abdominal organs. The digestive organs of most people are usually filled with toxicity, infections and other parasites, which easily penetrate the vessels and spread out into the reproductive organs, creating various problems. In addition, when filled with toxins and gas, the digestive organs create excessive pressure on the blood vessels and lymph leading to the reproductive organs, which results in poor circulation. So together, poor circulation, toxicity and infection result in related illnesses and sexual dysfunctions. Age also plays a big role in these dysfunctions simply because physical activity is reduced and toxicity levels increase.

Age and Prostate Problems

As a man gets older, the cells in his prostate are more likely to multiply, increasing the size of the gland. In modern theory it is believed that it is not the cells that multiply, but parasites taking the form of the cells. At the age of 30, a man has only 10 percent chance of having an enlarged prostate. At the age of 60 a man has more than 50 percent chance of having this problem, and more than 90 percent at age 85.

Do Not Be Ignorant

Most men are likely to ignore their prostate until it gives trouble. Unfortunately in modern Western society, the majority of prostates are trouble-makers to some degree. Many men are susceptible to the beginnings of prostatic hyperplasia, also known as enlarged prostate.

What Are the Symptoms of Prostate Trouble?

- Difficulty in starting to urinate
- Increased urinary frequency
- Nighttime trips to the bathroom
- Reduced force of volume of urination
- Sleep deprivation is common among men with prostate trouble.

How to Cleanse the Prostate and Improve Its Function

- Cleanse your whole digestive system (5-10 times) with FIR on the prostate area. Do parasite cleansing for at least 3 months.

- Start eating a healthy diet (read Book 4 in my series, *Healing through Cleansing Diet.*)
- Cleanse your small intestine (2-4 times).
- Cleanse your liver (3-5 times).
- Do cell cleansing for 2-3 weeks, three cycles.
- Maintain your colon cleansings and healthy lifestyle forever.

Therapeutic Benefits of Prostate Cleansing

- Rejuvenate your sex life
- Shrink the prostate to normal size
- Better urinary start, force, and volume
- Normalized urinary frequency
- Sleep with less interruption
- More efficient sleep
- Improved sexuality

SELF HELP: *PROSTATE RESTORATION*

Recommendations to restore normal prostate functions.

1. Cleanse your Large Intestine
2. Cleanse your Liver
3. Cleanse your Kidneys
4. Do not allow constipation and do not hold urination.
5. Drink enough fluids
6. Completely exclude spicy foods
7. Completely stay away from alcohol
8. Do "Deer exercise" 2 times per day

Urine Therapy

Urine Therapy is an ancient and an amazingly effective method.

In the modern technical and mechanical society, humans are detached from nature so not everyone is able to accept this type of therapy. If you are one of those people, you may discontinue reading this chapter. All procedures offered in our Center are very effective, and you can get great results without urine therapy. However, if you are open for something "new," want to know more and go deeper, you may continue reading.

What is Urine Therapy?

Urine Therapy is used for healing, maintenance or preventative purposes. The first question that comes to your mind is probably "How can my body's waste heal me?! We were always told that urine contains poisons, how can they be healthy?"

Urine develops from the blood, which filters through the kidneys. So basically, urine is your filtered blood, which has less toxicity than contaminated blood. Blood contamination occurs when the digestive system (stomach, small intestine and colon) are unclean. If the digestive system and the liver (the main blood filter) are clean, then the blood is also clean. So in this case, urine derived from clean blood becomes healing. It contains very little waste, and it carries complete information on all the problems and disorders in the body. For example, if you put some fresh urine on a cut or burn, the healing process will be much quicker.

Urine consumed orally, cleanses stomach walls, dissolves toxic mucus, works as a light laxative and diuretic, and cleanses blood vessels as well. Again, note that only urine derived from the clean system (after complete cleansing of the digestive system and liver) and good diet, has such strong healing qualities. Clean urine doesn't have bad smell and tastes just like water. Urine derived from an unclean system, smells bad, has a bad taste and doesn't have such strong healing powers. So, if you have cleansed your system, you may try to use urine internally and externally.

If you'd like to learn more about this therapy, you can easily find many books about it or information on the internet. Here I can give you some practical recommendations based on my personal experience:

1. Fresh urine can be drunk 1-5 times daily 2-8 oz (50-200 ml).
2. You must drink the whole amount without stopping (if you stopped, do not continue).
3. Drink a mid-portion of freshly released urine only. The first few drops may contain some bacteria, which got into urinary tract from the surface, and the last part may contain excess bile. So when you collect your urine, the first and last 1-2 oz. should not be collected.
4. You can drink urine from 2-3 a.m. to 8 p.m. Urine drunk between 2 a.m. and 5 a.m. has more healing information, so it is more healing.
5. Urine collected between 5 a.m. and 7 a.m. holds the most hormones. This part is recommended for those who have hormonal problems and imbalances.
6. Between 7 a.m. and 9 a.m. urine cures stomach disorders.
7. Throughout the day urine is a nutritious food supplement, carrying many nutrients and ALL amino acids. It is best to drink it one hour before the meal or 2-3 hours after the meal.

8. Externally, urine can be used for massage, baths or applied to wounds.
9. You can use fresh urine, or evaporated urine (to 1/2 or 1/4 of original amount) or even 3-5 day-old urine. For drinking use fresh urine. For external use, use old or evaporated urine. You may also drink evaporated urine 1-3 sips, 1-2 times per day.
10. Urine has been used externally to treat skin disorders.
11. Urine wraps are able to dissolve cysts/fibroids, heal burns, etc.
12. Fresh urine can be dropped in the eyes and ears or even to flush the nose and sinuses. By doing so, cataract, ear and sinus disease can be healed.
13. Fresh and evaporated urine can be used to rinse the mouth and throat. This kills bacteria in the gums and in the throat.
14. Fresh and evaporated urine can be used for small enemas to cleanse the lower part of the large intestine and rectum as well as to cure constipation, hemorrhoids, polyps and prostate related problems.
15. Urine can also be used during the fast. A urine fast in combination with cleansing procedures is the most effective way of fasting, and can be used to heal very serious illnesses, disorders and diseases.

More detailed information about the urine therapy, can be received during individual consultation by taking your individual health problems into consideration.

Sinus Cleansing

The Natural Way to Breathe Easy
Did you know that most people after age 30-40 can hold up
to 2 full cups of toxic mucus, infections, dust, pollen and
other substances of city air in their sinus cavity?

Did you know that all that dirt is the source of allergies,
asthma, colds, difficulty breathing, sinus pains, headaches,
ear infections, etc.?

All of it causes oxygen deprivation in result of which brain
functions, such as clear thinking, are disturbed.

One of the most common health complaints today seems to
be "sinuses." Millions of people take all kinds of drugs and
other remedies to relieve their symptoms when the solution
to their various nasal problems is literally right under their
noses.

The Source of the Problem

The sinuses are cavities just behind our noses that
connect the nose to the windpipe. These small but important
spaces in the front of our faces filter the air we breathe,
removing a wide variety of harmful substances. This filtering
action protects the lungs from airborne dust, microscopic
lifeforms such as mites, pollen, pollution and various other
things that are best removed before they reach the lungs.
Because of this, and for other reasons, the sinus cavities can

become inflamed and clogged with a waste product called mucous. (Sinusitis is the proper term for this inflammation.)

What Problems Does Sinusitis Cause?

As many people have found out the hard way, this excess mucus makes it difficult for air to flow through the nostrils. This causes the lungs to work harder which in turn puts a physical strain on the heart. This also creates an oxygen deficiency for the organs of the body, particularly the brain. When people can't breathe through their nostrils they tend to breathe through their mouths. Breathing through our mouths doesn't protect our lungs and bronchus from infections, and it doesn't warm up the air enough.

The heating and air conditioning systems we so enjoy - at home and in the car - are efficient mechanisms for the spreading of airborne viruses and bacteria. When these organisms reach mucous-clogged sinuses, they find the perfect environment (and food) for their growth and development. This situation can easily lead to the inflammation of the sinuses.

The body certainly does not sustain this waste, so as soon as it is created it begins to decay. As it accumulates in the sinuses it causes problems for the eyes, ears and your brain. The simple act of breathing brings some of these contaminants passed the sinuses, and into the lungs and bronchus creating more mucous there. The side effects of sinusitis can be serious; people who suffer from sinusitis, also experience many other related problems.

The Real Culprit

But the contaminants in the air we breathe are not the only cause of sinus problems. Something much more common, and completely unexpected, can be at the root of a great number of nasal problems. The main cause of sinusitis is found in our diet. Foods such as dairy products, white flour, refined grains, sweets, processed foods, etc. can react badly with our personal chemistries and cause the body to generate excessive amounts of mucous. Unfortunately this excessive mucous ends up in various organs throughout the body, particularly the colon. This kind of mucous is a perfect site for the beginnings of cancer.

Can Someone Who Has Sinusitis Be Treated?

It is almost impossible to cure sinusitis with pharmaceuticals. Symptoms can be alleviated, but that is about it. By themselves, our bodies are not able to completely get rid of the sometimes large amounts of excess mucus that accumulate throughout the body. The good news is that alternative or natural methods work very effectively, and can help not only the sinuses, but the rest of the body as well. The approach outlined below is easier, less expensive, and has no side effects except proper weight loss and improved health.

What Should I do To Get Rid Of Sinusitis Problems Completely?

1. If the problem is not very severe.

The most important first step is to cleanse your large intestine (colon) of wastes that have built up there over the years. This one organ is the largest storehouse of toxic mucus and other toxic substances, and must be cleaned before the rest of this program can be effective.

It would be very wise to do Stomach cleansing in conjunction with Sinus cleansing since mucous can accumulate there as well.

At the Koyfman Whole Body Cleansing we have specialized equipment that allows us to clean toxic mucus, viruses and bacterias from the sinuses. We also use an organic solution which helps eliminate wastes from the sinuses and disinfects them.

It is important to remove from your diet all foods, which cause your body to produce mucus.

In my book *"Healing Through Cleansing 2"* you can learn what you can do at home to your sinuses clean and healthy on daily basis, as well as different remedies for quick relieve of sinus pains and discomforts.

2. In more serious cases,

it will be necessary to do cleansing down to the cellular level. This cleansing includes: the cleansing of the **small intestine, lymph cleansing and juice fasting**.

If you go through this program, you will relieve not only your sinusitis problem, but many other disorders and health problems. Cleansing will improve your vision, hearing and mental clarity!

"...I have chronic sinusitis for over 3 years. Doctors are feeding me antibiotics, but it only makes the problem worse. When I started trying Dr. Koyfman's methods, I felt a tremendous difference right away. Together with other cleansing procedures and dietary recommendations, this cleanse is very effective. I can finally breathe through my nose, which I forgot how to do a long time ago..."

James N.

Maintenance
Program

"Do not lose the ground
you have gained"

What Have You Achieved after Completing the Eight Steps of the Program?

If in the past you have had a complete cleansing course, or even part of the cleansing program, you are already beginning to notice great improvements in your health. You are definitely interested in maintaining and multiplying your achievement.

1.   You feel stronger.
2.   You have more energy.
3.   Your immune system is stronger and not wasting energy on neutralizing toxins.
4.   Your skin looks and feels better.
5.   Your breathing is easier and cleaner (no odor).
6.   Your large intestine eliminates regularly.
7.   You significantly reduced your health age and the health problems which come with age.
8.   And much more.

What Is Important to Remember?

The health improvement you have achieved carries with it **no warranty to protect forever** from disorders, illnesses, tiredness, and other problems. Why? We all live in

212

a poisoned world, so our bodies are being polluted continually and constantly. **There is a mistaken opinion that the system can clean itself completely by itself, but if this were possible humans would never get ill and never die.**

Negative emotions can change the chemical make up of the best food products, turning them into poison. Negative emotions also weaken the functions of all eliminating organs. This results in additional pollution of the body.

Food is very important for all of us. Many people eat three times a day. So let's take a look at how the body is polluted from food. The level of pollution from food depends on many factors:

1. Whether it is organic or regular.
2. Whether it is fruit or meat.
3. Whether you have strong or weak digestion.
4. Whether or not you feel hungry when you eat.
5. How you chew your food.
6. The volume you eat
7. The time when you eat, late evening or allowing time to digest the food
8. Whether it is processed food or fresh.

Because we cannot take everything into consideration, let's look at some of the moderating factors. All the volume (100%) of each meal can be divided into three parts.

1. Since the body can assimilate or digest only liquid, therefore, only 15-25% of the volume eaten will be digested. **Explanation:** Juice made in a juice maker (excluding watermelon, cucumber, and other especially juicy products) may reach one-third (30%) of the full volume, however, this extent of

"digestion" or pulverization will not be possible in the presence of poor chewing, bad or missing teeth, or a weak digestive system. So the body gets less juice from eating food than the juice maker gets.

2. The second and third parts together make up approximately 75-85% of the volume eaten. The second part, mostly fiber at 25-40%, is eliminated after 12-36 hours by the work of the colon. The other 25% to 35% of the second part stays longer and cannot be eliminated by colon work alone but depends on the help of pressure from new material pushing, and gravity pulling, on the material inside the colon. This longer time period allows for the process of putrefaction and decay, and the immune system must waste energy to neutralize the poisons produced.

3. The third part is excessive fat, mucous, and non-digestible protein, amounting to 3-10% and more. This is encrusted material that sticks to the colon wall and stays in the system a long time or maybe forever. It becomes dehydrated and pressed to the walls. In time, with lack of oxygen, and with warmth and darkness, this material begins putrefaction and decay, creating an environment for parasites to develop. **If you do preventive Colon Cleansing once in two to four weeks, this will save you from accumulating poisons and parasites.**

Can Regular Preventive Colon Cleansing Completely Protect a Person from All Health Problems?

Even though you try to follow all suggestions and rules of good diet, healthy lifestyle, and cleansing procedures, in reality it is rare that you will do it perfectly. Sometimes you will experience headache, tiredness, colds, stomach discomfort, etc. It is very important **to notice the feeling of he beginning of these disorders,** before they develop.

If you want to solve the problem quickly, you have to stop eating for three to five days, and every other day do some Colon Cleansing. This will quickly help to increase the effectiveness of the immune system and eliminate the problem. The disease will not be able to go deep into the body and do its damage.

We can call them **entrance disorders** if we catch them when they enter, and if you take correct measures in time you will not allow these problems to go inside the system. But if you delay and allow the problem to develop, it can go deep into organs and tissues and cells, and then the problem will continue developing from inside.

Such disorders we can call **internal or chronic disorders.** To solve these problem is very difficult. If they continue a long time these chronic disorders can accumulate and transform into serious illnesses.

Tips to Remember

1. Do not insult others, and try to understand and forgive those who insult you. Insults could be lessons for your own improvement.

2. Try to follow all suggestions about the cleansing diet.

3. Every day do exercises for spine, joints, internal organs, and the endocrine system. If you do your exercises correctly together with outdoor walking, you will activate the **process of cell feeding and cleansing.**

4. Cleanse regularly your colon once in two to four weeks.

5. If you feel the first sign of disorders, stop eating for one to five days, and every other day cleanse your colon.

6. Do Small Intestine Cleansing every three months.

7. Do Complex Liver Cleansing one or two times per year.

8. More often than usual, do specific cleansings which manage your individual problems.

9. If you are interested to get the highest level of health, do a long fast for 2-4 weeks every year, strictly following the instructions in the chapter on cell cleansing.

Unique Method of Colon Rejuvenation, 95 pgs; $12.
Our bodies need constant help eliminating toxic
substances which enter the system every day.
Daily practice of the rising and restroom
exercises described in this book strengthens
colon muscles so that, with time, elimination
will accompany each meal and eject more
toxins than are retained. Also included are
principles and recipes for healthy eating, raw
meals, and safe cooking technology.

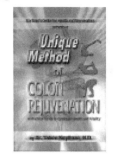

Deep Internal Body Cleansing, 172 pgs.
If you search for healing and real health, then
here you will find answers to your questions
Here is information about toxicity and the
immune system, healthy eating and eliminating
parasites. Here are answers to help you resist
hurtful cravings and negative emotions. You
really can get health and gain energy through
cleansing your body.

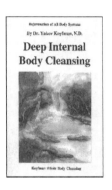

Healing Through Cleansing - Book 1, 112
pgs; $12.
Every day, toxic substances enter our bodies
from the various chemical and biological
contaminants in our environment. Additionally,
toxins form within us due to poor dietary habits,
stress, aging, and harmful bacteria that populate
our bodies. Our excretory organs can't cope
with such a large amount of work and need
constant, conscious support. How can you help

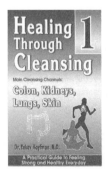

your main excretory organs become free of toxins, bacteria,
and infections? You will find the answers in the pages of this
and subsequent books in this Koyfman Series.

Healing Through Cleansing - Book 2, 102 pgs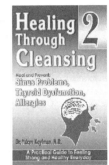
In many ways our health depends on the health of
organs located in the head and neck regions: the
brain, thyroid gland, eyes, salivary glands, ears,
nose and sinuses, throat, tongue, teeth and gums.
The contemporary American diet usually includes
a large number of mucus-forming foods that
result in the generation of mucus throughout the
body. Excess mucus settles throughout the body,
especially in the head and neck organs, giving rise to a number
of ailments in these organs.

Healing Through Cleansing - Book 3, 120 pgs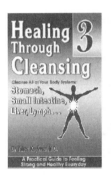
The abdominal area is the kitchen of our bodies.
How well or poorly this kitchen functions
depends on whether we feed our system with
nutrients or poison our system with toxicity. If
your abdominal kitchen produces nutrients, you
are getting health; if your kitchen produces
poison, you are getting disease. How can you help
your abdominal organs to become more healthy
and free of toxins and to sustain the health of your entire body?
You will find the answers in the pages of this book.

Healing Through Cleansing Diet - Book 4, 112 pgs

"To get the best results in the healing process, it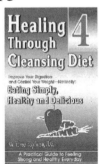
is not enough to find a skilled teacher who can
guide you along the path. It is also very
important that the student be open-minded to
new information and ready to work," says Dr.
Yakov Koyfman, N.D. A healthy diet gives to
the system not only nutrients but also help to
clean and heal the body. To make your diet
healthy, you need to learn the things in this
book.